J. Richard Smith • Jeremiah Healy • Giuseppe Del Priore (Eds)

Atlas of Staging in Gynecological Cancer

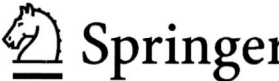

J. Richard Smith, MB, ChB, MD, FRCOG
Consultant Gynaecological Oncologist
West London Gynaecological Cancer Centre
Hammersmith & Queen Charlotte's Hospital
London
UK

Jeremiah Healy, MRCP, FRCR
Consultant Radiologist
Chelsea and Westminster Hospital
London
UK

Giuseppe Del Priore, MD, MPH
Vice President Research
New York Downtown Hospital
New York
USA

British Library Cataloguing in Publication Data
Atlas of staging in gynecological cancer
   1. Generative organs, Female – Cancer – Atlases 2. Tumors – Classification
   I. Smith, J. Richard II. Healy, Jeremiah III. Del Priore, Giuseppe
   616.9'9465

ISBN-13: 978-1-84628-433-5   e-ISBN-13: 978-1-84628-434-2

Printed on acid-free paper

9 8 7 6 5 4 3 2 1

Springer Science+Business Media
springer.com

Contents

Acknowledgements vii

Editors and Contributors ix

Cervical Cancer   J.A. Lacombe, G. Del Priore and J. Hillier 1

Vaginal Cancer   M.K. Guess and A. Sohaib 6

Vulval Carcinoma   S. Ghaem-Maghami, A. McIndoe, E. Moskovic and A. Sohaib 9

Endometrial Cancer   A. Wang, K.M. Hartzfeld and M. Hughes 15

Ovarian Cancer   S. Shahabi and A. Sohaib 20

Gestational Trophoblastic Disease   K. Sieunarine, J.R. Smith, A. Aylwin and A. Mitchell 25

Acknowledgements

The FIGO staging system (†) is reproduced by courtesy of the International Federation of Gynecology and Obstetrics, previously published in the International Journal of Gynecology and Obstetrics, Vol. 83, Sup. 1, October 2003.

The American Joint Committee on Cancer surgical staging system (‡) is used with the permission of the American Joint Committee on Cancer (AJCC), Chicago, Illinois, USA. The original source for this material is the AJCC Cancer Staging Manual, Sixth Edition (2002), edited by F.L. Greene, D.L. Page, I.D. Fleming et al, published by Springer New York, www.springer.com

Illustrations by courtesy of Health Press Ltd., Abingdon, UK, taken from the publications Fast Facts Gynaecological Oncology, Fast Facts Breast Cancer, and Patient Pictures Breast Cancer.

Editors

J.R. Smith, MB, ChB, MD, FRCOG
Consultant Gynaecological Oncologist
West London Gynaecological Cancer Centre
Hammersmith & Queen Charlotte's Hospital
London, UK

J. Healy, MRCP, FRCR
Consultant Radiologist
Chelsea & Westminster Hospital
London, UK

Giuseppe Del Priore, MD, MPH
Vice President Research
NY Downtown Hospital
NY-Presbyterian Healthcare
New York, USA

Contributors

Anthony Aylwin, MRCP, FRCR
Consultant Radiologist
Charing Cross Hospital
London, UK

S. Ghaem-Maghami, PhD, MRCOG
Consultant Gynaecological Oncologist
Hammersmith & Queen Charlotte's Hospital
London, UK

Marsha Guess, MD
Yale University School of Medicine
Connecticut, USA

Kimberly M. Hartzfeld, MD
New York Downtown Hospital
New York, USA

Julia Hillier, MRCP, FRCR
Consultant Radiologist
Chelsea & Westminster Hospital
London, UK

Michael Hughes, MRCP, FRCR
Consultant Radiologist
Charing Cross Hospital
London, UK

Julia A. Lacombe, MD
University of Vermont
College of Medicine
Vermont, USA

A. McIndoe PhD, FRCS, FRCCOG
Consultant Gynaecological Oncologist
Hammersmith and Queen Charlotte's Hospital
London, UK

Adam Mitchell, FRCS, FRCR
Consultant Radiologist
Charing Cross Hospital
London, UK

E. Moskovic, FRCP, FRCR
Consultant Radiologist
Royal Marsden Hospital
London, UK

Shohreh Shahabi, MD
Montefiore Medical Center
New York, USA

Aslam Sohaib, MRCP, FRCR
Consultant Radiologist
Royal Marsden Hospital
London, UK

K. Sieunarine, MRCOG
Research Fellow
Chelsea & Westminster Hospital
London, UK

Andrea S. Wang, MD
Columbia University
College of Physicians & Surgeons
New York, USA

CERVICAL CANCER

J.A. Lacombe, G. Del Priore and J. Hillier

Introduction

Approximately 12 000 women were newly diagnosed with cervical cancer in the USA in 2003.[1] Although cervical cancer remains a leading killer of women worldwide, the incidence in the USA represents a significant decrease, mainly attributable to the widespread implementation of Pap test screening. The Pap smear is designed for detecting pre-invasive disease of the cervix. This allows treatment to be initiated prior to the development of cancer.[2]

Human papillomavirus (HPV) is a sexually transmitted virus associated with cervical dysplasia and invasive cancer. Low-risk HPV types, such as 6 and 11, are associated with cervical intraepithelial neoplasia (CIN) I and condyloma. High-risk types of HPV, such as types 16, 18, 31, 33 and 35, are observed in association with high-grade dysplasia or cervical cancer. HPV DNA can be detected in close to 100% of patients with invasive cervical cancer. Although the prevalence of HPV in some populations approaches 30–90%, only a small number of these women go on to develop cervical cancer.[2]

The overwhelming majority of cervical carcinomas have historically been of squamous cell histology. However, with improvement in the diagnosis and treatment of pre-invasive cervical cancer the percentage of adenocarcinomas has steadily risen from the 1970s to the present. In 1996 24% of diagnosed cervical cancer was adenocarcinoma representing a twofold rise in incidence from 1973.[3] The diagnosis, treatment and prognosis of both histological subgroups appear to be similar.

Staging

Because the majority of the cases of cervical cancer worldwide are in women living in underdeveloped countries, staging systems for cervical cancer have been clinically based. Staging procedures have accordingly been geared towards technologies available within these countries.

The International Federation of Gynecology and Obstetrics (Federation Internationale Gynecologique Obstetrique or FIGO) along with the World Health Organization last revised its staging system in 1995.[4] The FIGO staging (Table 2.1) system is based upon a thorough clinical examination, chest X-ray, intravenous pyelogram, cystoscopy, proctoscopy and barium enema as indicated. The physical examination should include abdominal, pelvic, rectovaginal and lymph node examinations. Examination under anaesthesia is strongly recommended because of the added benefits of muscular relaxation and inter-examiner correlation.[5] If up-to-date imaging methods are available such as magnetic resonance imaging (MRI) and positron emission tomography (PET) scanning, an examination under anaesthesia EUA may not be needed for treatment planning.

According to the FIGO staging guidelines, a major distinction exists between micro-invasion stage IA disease versus macroscopic stage IB disease. Micro-invasive disease is further delineated as stage IA1, with stromal invasion less than 3 mm in depth with a maximum horizontal spread of 7 mm and stage IA2, defined as stromal invasion up to 5 mm with the same horizontal spread up to 7 mm on a single histology slide. Micro-invasive cervical cancer is generally diagnosed upon cone biopsy following an abnormal Pap smear and colposcopy. Stage IA disease generally carries an extremely good prognosis. However, these distinctions are of extreme importance in the determination of which patients can be treated conservatively versus those who require more aggressive treatment.[5,6]

The American Joint Committee on Cancer (AJCC) has established a TNM (tumour, node, metastasis) classification system based on the same clinical staging information as FIGO. According to the AJCC, the T stages correspond to the FIGO stages. The AJCC recommends that surgical and pathologic findings be recorded as a final pathologic (TMN) disease stage, but should not change the clinical FIGO stage.

Controversy exists regarding surgical staging for cervical cancer. In 1980 the Gynecologic Oncology Group (GOG) reported a greater than 30% risk of para-aortic lymph node metastasis in patients with locally advanced cervical cancer, i.e. stages IB2–III.[7] Many authors have advocated lymphadenectomy in cervical cancer for prognostic information as well as to assist in the planning of radiation fields.[5,8] The advent of laparoscopy has made this procedure less morbid, thereby renewing interest in surgical staging.[8] However, a consistent survival benefit has not been demonstrated.[5]

Imaging studies and cervical cancer

Lymphangiography can be used to assign staging in the FIGO system. A computed tomography (CT) scan, MRI and a PET scan cannot be included in the FIGO staging procedure, but certainly change treatment decisions when available. These imaging studies are useful in accurately determining the extent of disease spread in order to tailor treatment for patients with cervical cancer. Advances in imaging could improve the accuracy of staging cervical cancer by facilitating the detection of lymph node and distant organ metastases. This procedure is rarely used when the modern alternatives described below are available because it is painful and operator dependent leading to questionable reliability.[9]

Lymphangiography

Lymphangiography involves injecting a contrast dye into the lymphatic system prior to X-ray imaging. Normal lymph nodes appear opaque and lymph nodes with neoplastic cells do not. The cervix has predictable drainage to local lymph nodes and is well suited to lymphangiography.

The dorsal pedal lymphatics are identified using a visible blue dye. The identified lymphatic channels are then canalized and radiographic contrast injected with direct observation of the pelvic nodes at risk. The reported sensitivities are in the range of 28–83% and the specificities are in the range of 47–100%.[9]

Computed tomography

CT scans are completed with the use of a 360° X-ray beam and computer reproduction of images. These scans allow for multiplanar cross-sectional and three-dimensional views of body organs and tissues.

Imaging studies and cervical cancer *continued*

In the staging of cervical cancer, CT may be unofficially substituted for an intravenous pyelogram in the evaluation of ureteral obstruction. In addition, CT scans may provide information regarding tumour size, lymph node enlargement and the presence of distant metastases. CT and MRI have comparable accuracies in determining lymph node metestases in cervical carcinoma of 85-95%.[10] Meta-analysis of published studies confirmed that CT and MRI performed to a similar degree of accuracy in the detection of lymph node metestases and slightly better than lymphangiography.[11] A finding of enlarged lymph nodes on CT scanning has a specificity of 93%, but a positive predictive value of only 39%.[9,10]

Enlarged lymph nodes or evidence of metastatic disease on a CT scan warrant further investigation with other imaging or biopsy.

Magnetic resonance imaging

MRI employs radio frequency pulses as opposed to ionizing radiation for mapping internal structures. Although MRI and CT scanning are comparable in their ability for determining lymph node status, MRI is far superior to CT scanning in soft tissue contrast resolution. MRI provides a detailed survey of pelvic anatomy and has proven useful for determining tumour size, the depth of invasion and parametrial involvement and identifying bladder and rectal extension. Several authors have demonstrated the accuracy of MRI for pre-treatment staging to be greater than 90%.[5,9–13] The primary use of MRI appears to be in assisting in the determination of a patient's operability.

Positron emission tomography

Through the use of labelled isotopes, 2-[F-18]flouro-2-deoxy-D-glucose(18 FDG PET) scanning provides a functional assessment of glycolytic activity within a patient's body. In this way, FDG-PET is a non-invasive method of detecting metastatic disease in cancer. Its utility due to a high specificity and sensitivity has been demonstrated in cancers of the lung, head and neck and oesophagus. The use of PET scanning in cervical cancer is thought to be more accurate for the detection of lymph node spread than CT scanning or MRI. The sensitivity of PET scanning for lymph node status in cervical cancer has been shown to be between 75 and 90%. Most importantly, the negative predictive value is over 90%.[9,14,15]

The role of PET scanning in the diagnosis of recurrent cervical cancer and, specifically, the determination of appropriate candidates for total pelvic exenteration is currently under investigation and appears promising. Evolving technologies have combined PET scanning with CT scanning or MRI in order to combine an anatomical image with the functional PET scanning result. Further investigation is needed into specific uses for this novel technology.

Lymphatic mapping

Sentinal lymph node identification is a technique that involves a peri-tumoral injection of a short-lived radioactive substance and/or a blue dye that is then transported by the lymphatic channels to the sentinel lymph node. This modality has been routinely used in melanoma, breast cancer, penile cancer and vulvar cancer. Larger trials need to be performed in order to assess the sensitivity, specificity and safety of sentinel node detection in cervical cancer.[16]

Treatment

The treatment of cervical cancer is individualized to each patient based upon her stage and concomitant medical problems. Treatment may include surgery, radiation, chemotherapy or a combination of all three modalities.

Surgical management

Because the risk of nodal involvement in early micro-invasive cervical cancer (stage IA1) is less than 1%, patients with stage IA1 disease can be treated simply with a total abdominal hysterectomy performed via the abdominal, vaginal or laparoscopic route.[16] In young patients with a desire to preserve fertility, a cone biopsy may be considered therapeutic. However, even with stromal invasion of ≤3 mm, a patient must be counselled as to her small but real risk of residual disease after a cone biopsy. In addition, many practitioners would recommend total hysterectomy at the completion of childbearing.[5,16,17] With stromal invasion of up to 5 mm (stage IA2) the risk of lymph node metastasis increases to 6–7%.[16] This is generally felt to be an unacceptably high risk and simple hysterectomy an under-treatment. Radical hysterectomy with pelvic and para-aortic lymph node dissection is the recommended surgical procedure for patients who are medically stable with disease confined to the cervix and upper vagina (stages IA2, IB and IIA).[5] Radical hysterectomy allows for sampling and removal of the cervix, uterus, parametrial and paracervical tissues and upper vagina. Tumour volume may be used as a determinant of surgical respectability. The formula for calculation of the volume of a cervical tumour is $D^3 \times {}^\pi/_3$ [5].

Novel surgical procedures for early stage cervical cancer are available and may in the future change the standard of care. In young women interested in retaining the possibility of childbearing, a radical trachelectomy appears to be both a safe and effective treatment. This can be performed abdominally or vaginally. The advent of minimally invasive surgery has brought about interest in a variant of the classic Shauta procedure, where a radical vaginal hysterectomy can be performed with laparoscopic lymph node dissection. In addition, a total laparoscopic radical hysterectomy has also been developed.[17]

A small percentage of women with recurrent cervical cancer may be candidates for pelvic exenteration. Total exenteration involves surgical resection of the pelvic viscera including the bladder and rectosigmoid colon. This procedure carries with it a high morbidity and mortality rate and a 5-year survival rate of approximately 20–65%. Patient selection and pre-operative counselling are crucial to the success of this operation.[18]

Radiation therapy

Patients with advanced stage (stages IIB, III and IVA) cervical cancer are generally not considered to be surgical candidates. These patients have been traditionally treated with external pelvic irradiation and brachytherapy combined with chemotherapy sensitization.[5,16] In addition, post-surgical patients with high-risk features on their final pathology should receive radiation therapy and/or chemotherapy. The combined modalities of surgery and radiation lead to an increase in morbidity that may be unacceptably high. An ongoing GOG trial is investigating whether patients with bulky local tumours (stage IB2) should be treated up front with radiation because of their likelihood of requiring post-operative radiation.[19] In addition, patients of any stage whose medical conditions preclude surgery should be referred for radiation therapy.

Chemotherapy
In 1999 two large randomized prospective studies concluded that chemotherapy administered along with radiation significantly improved survival compared to radiation alone.[16,20] As a result the standard of care has shifted to treatment involving concurrent chemotherapy with radiation therapy.[15] Patients with poor performance status, co-morbid medical conditions or metastatic disease need to be evaluated on a case-by-case basis as to the additional benefits of radiation. Chemotherapy is indicated in the treatment of metastatic (stage IVB) and extra-pelvic recurrences of cervical cancer. Although multiple chemotherapeutic regimens have shown activity against cervical cancer with initial response rates as high as 80%, the response rates are generally in the order of 20% in previously treated patients.[5]

Follow Up
Patients are reviewed 3–4 monthly for 2 years and then 6 monthly for the next 3 years. Most practitioners will then undertake annual review thereafter. Review should comprise examination and vaginal vault cytology.

References

1. *Cancer Facts and Figures*. The American Cancer Society; 2003.
2. Cannistra S, Niloff JM. Cancer of the uterine cervix. *N Engl J Med* 1996; **334**: 1030–7.
3. Smith HO *et al*. The rising incidence of adenocarcinoma relative to squamous cell carcinoma of the uterine cervix in the United States – a 24 year population-based study. *Gynecol Oncol* 2000; **78**: 97–105.
4. Creaseman WT. New gynecologic cancer staging. *Gynecol Oncol* 1995; **58**: 157.
5. Hoskins W, Perez CA, Young RC. *Principles and Practice of Gynecologic Oncology*. 2000.
6. Creasman WT. Stage IA cancer of the cervix: finally some resolution of definition and treatment. *Gynecol Oncol* 1999; **74**: 163–4.
7. Lagasse LD *et al*. Results and complications of operative staging in cervical cancer: experience of the Gynecologic Oncology Group. *Gynecol Oncol* 1980; **9**: 90.
8. Sonoda Y *et al*. Prospective evaluation of surgical staging of advanced cervical cancer via a laparoscopic extraperitoneal approach. *Gynecol Oncol* 2003; **91**: 326–31.
9. Follen M *et al*. Imaging in cervical cancer. *Cancer* 2003; **98**(9 Suppl): 2028–38.
10. Kim SH *et al*. Preoperative staging of uterine cervical carcinoma: comparison of CT and MRI in 99 patients. *J Comput Assist Tomogr* 1993; **17**: 633–40.
11. Subak LL *et al*. Cervical carcinoma: computed tomography and magnetic resonance imaging for preoperative staging. *Obstet Gynecol* 1995; **86**: 43–50.
12. Narayan K *et al*. A comparison of MRI and PET scanning in surgically staged loco-regionally advanced cervical cancer: potential impact on treatment. *Int J Gynecol Cancer* 2001; **11**: 263–71.
13. Kerr IG *et al*. Positron emission tomography for the evaluation of metastases in patients with carcinoma of the cervix: a retrospective review. *Gynecol Oncol* 2000; **81**: 477–80.
14. Grisbey PW, Herzog TJ. Current management of patients with invasive cervical carcinoma. *Clin Obstetr Gynecol* 2001; **44**: 531–7.
15. Herzog TJ. New approaches for the management of cervical cancer. *Gynecol Oncol* 2003; **90**: S22–7.
16. Disai PJ, Creasman WT. *Clinical Gynecologic Oncology*. 2002.
17. Disai P, Kellner JR. Protocol GOG-0201: treatment of patients with stage IB2 carcinoma of the cervix: a randomized comparison of radical hysterectomy and tailored chemo-radiation. 2003.
18. Rose PG *et al*. Concurrent cisplatin-based radiotherapy and chemotherapy for locally advanced cervical cancer. *N Engl J Med* 1999; **340**: 1144–53.

CARCINOMA OF THE CERVIX

† The FIGO staging system

FIGO Stage	0	1	IA	IA1	IA2	IB	IB1	IB2	II	IIA	IIB
	Carcinoma *in situ* and intra-epithelial carcinoma	Carcinoma is strictly confined to the cervix	Invasive cancer identified only microscopically, all gross lesions, even with superficial invasion, are stage IB cancers; invasion is limited to measured stromal invasion with a maximum depth of 5 mm and no wider than 7 mm	Measured invasion of stroma no greater than 3 mm in depth and no wider than 7 mm	Measured invasion of stroma greater than 3 mm and no greater than 5 mm in depth and no wider than 7 mm	Clinical lesions confined to the cervix or pre-clinical lesions greater than stage IA	Clinical lesions no greater than 4 cm in size	Clinical lesions greater than 4 cm in size	The carcinoma extends beyond the cervix, but has not extended on to the pelvic wall: the carcinoma involves the vagina, but not as far as the lower third	No obvious parametrial involvement	Obvious parametrial involvement

‡ American Joint Committee on Cancer surgical staging system

AJCC Stage	T	Tis		T1a	T1a1	T1a2	T1b	T1b1	T1b2		T2a	T2b
	N											
	M											

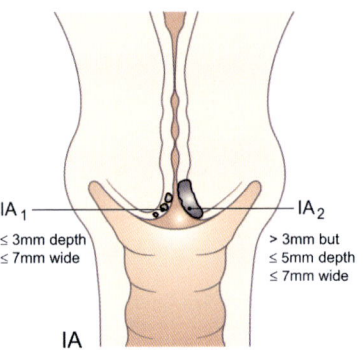

IA₁ — ≤ 3mm depth, ≤ 7mm wide

IA₂ — > 3mm but ≤ 5mm depth, ≤ 7mm wide

IA

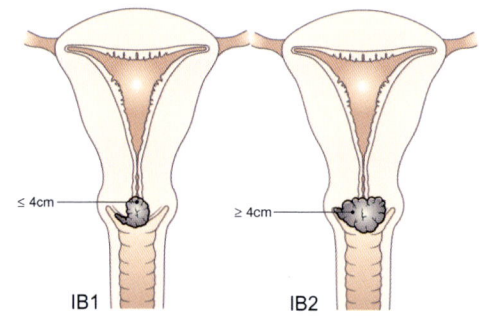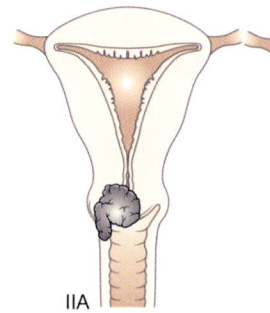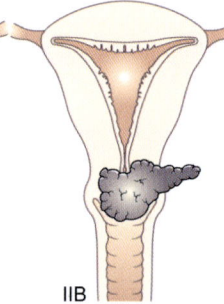

≤ 4cm — IB1

≥ 4cm — IB2

IIA

IIB

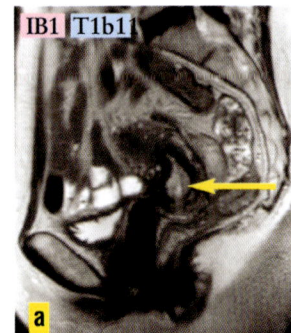

IB1 | T1b1

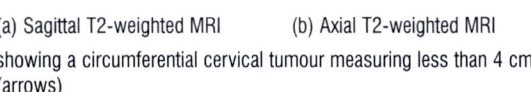

(a) Sagittal T2-weighted MRI (b) Axial T2-weighted MRI

showing a circumferential cervical tumour measuring less than 4 cm (arrows)

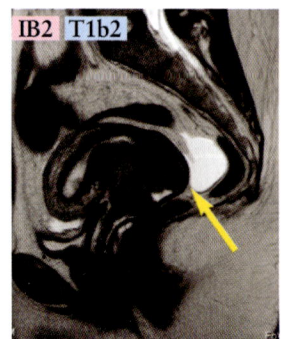

IB2 | T1b2

Sagittal T2-weighted MRI showing a bulky cervical carcinoma measuring more than 4 cm. Note that the tumour is not invading the posterior aspect of the vagina (arrow).

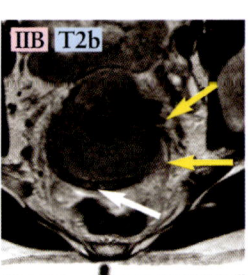

IIB | T2b

Axial T2-weighted MRI showing a large cervical tumour showing extension into the parametrium (yellow arrows). The low-signal normal cervical stroma is completely absent. Note that the tumour is not invading the posterior wall of the vagina (white arrow).

III

The carcinoma has extended on to the pelvic wall, on rectal examination there is no cancer-free space between the tumour and the pelvic wall, the tumour involves the lower third of the vagina; all cases with a hydronephrosis or non-functioning kidney should be included, unless they are known to be due to another cause

IIIA

No extension on to the pelvic wall, but involvement of the lower third of the vagina

IIIB

Extension on to the pelvic wall or hydronephrosis or non-functioning kidney

IV

The carcinoma has extended beyond the true pelvis or has clinically involved the mucosa of the bladder or rectum

IVA

Spread of the growth to adjacent organs

IVB

Spread to distant organs

| T3a | T1, 2, 3a, 3b N1 | T4 any N | any T any N M1 |

IIIA | T3a

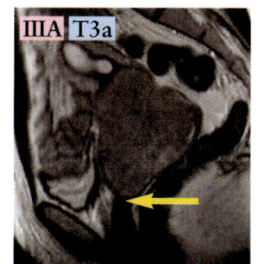

Sagittal T2-weighted MRI showing a bulky cervical tumour extending into the lower third of the vagina (arrow).

IIIA | T3a

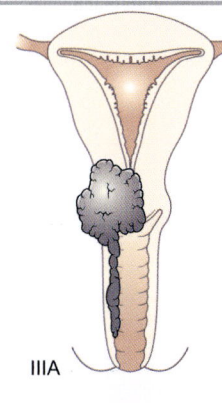

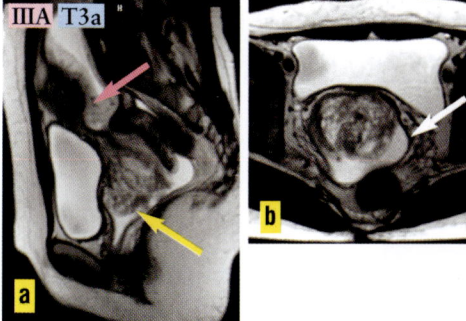

(a) Sagittal T2-weighted MRI (b) axial T2-weighted MRI

showing a mixed-signal tumour of the anterior lip of the cervix extending into the lower third of the vagina (yellow arrow). Note that the low signal of the vaginal wall is intact (white arrow). The high signal within the uterus is due to concurrent pregnancy (pink arrow).

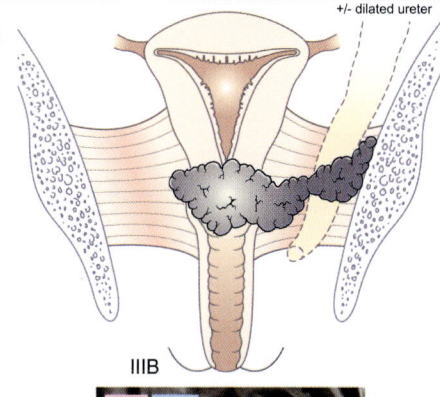

IIIA

+/- dilated ureter

IIIB

IIIB | T3b

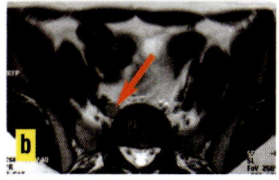

a

b

(a) Sagittal and (b) axial T2-weighted MRI showing a bulky cervical tumour (yellow arrow) with no evidence of extension into the parametrium. However, a right iliac lymph node metastasis is noted (red arrow)

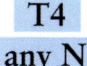

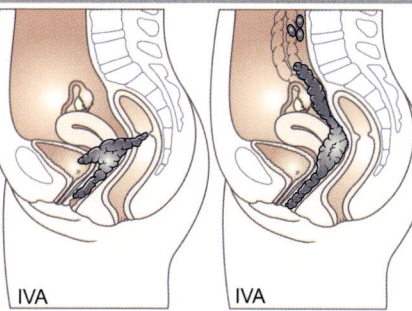

IVA

IVA

IVA | T4, any N

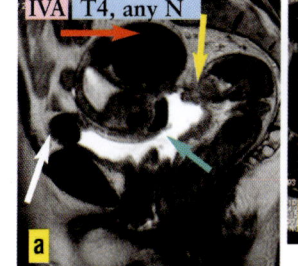

a

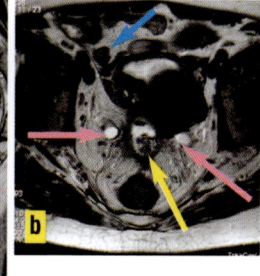

b

(a) Sagittal and (b) axial T2-weighted images of the pelvis showing a cervical carcinoma (yellow arrow) that has eroded into the bladder causing a large vagino-vesical fistula (green arrow). Gas is seen in the bladder and the vagina (white arrow). Note the posterior wall fibroids within the uterus (red arrow). There is bilateral hydronephrosis (pink arrows). Note the right external iliac lymph node (blue arrow).

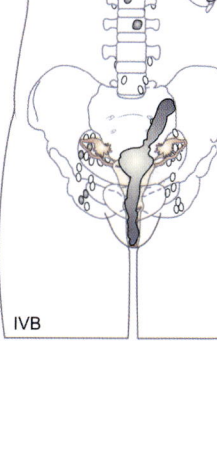

IVB

VAGINAL CANCER

M.K. Guess and A. Sohaib

Introduction

Primary vaginal cancer is a rare malignancy, representing approximately 2% of gynaecological malignancies and only approximately 0.1–0.2% of all cancers.[1] The vast majority (85%) of vaginal cancers are of squamous origin: however, adenocarcinomas, clear cell carcinomas, melanomas and sarcomas are infrequently identified. Although secondary vaginal carcinomas are more common than primary tumours, the keen pathologist can distinguish between the two using conventional standards. Specifically, a primary vaginal cancer should be diagnosed only when the cervix is uninvolved with an obvious focus of tumour origin in the vagina. When an apparent malignancy is found in the vagina and these conditions are not met, secondary vaginal cancer should be considered. Secondary vaginal cancer may represent an extension from a cervical cancer or metastatic disease from a uterine, ovarian, vulvar, bladder or colon primary tumour.

Staging

Many authors deem the stage of disease at the time of diagnosis as the most important prognostic factor. However, other factors, such as the initial tumour volume, extent of vaginal tissue involvement, histological grade and lymphatic involvement, may also impact on survival.[2–5] According to the accepted standard of the staging of the International Federation of Gynecology and Obstetrics (Federation Internationale Gynecologique Obstetrique or FIGO)[6] (Table 3.1) vaginal cancers are staged clinically. A thorough history and physical examination should be coupled with diagnostic studies so that local and distant disease spread can be readily identified and treatment can be tailored to the individual.

Stage 0 is carcinoma *in situ* or high grade vaginal intra-epithelial neoplasia (VAIN3). The slightly imprecise nature of the margins of the vagina make the staging more arbitrary. As a result the staging of this tumour involves close collaboration between gynaecologist, radiologist and pathologist. The definitions of stages 0–IV are shown in the figures on page 9.

Supplementary diagnostic studies for clinical staging

In addition to a pelvic and rectovaginal digital examination, ancillary tests should be performed in order to ensure accurate diagnosis and staging of the disease. The routine work-up should include a cervical cytological smear and a thorough inspection of the vagina, including colposcopy and biopsy and an endometrial biopsy is also usually indicated.

1. Computed tomography (CT) scans. A CT scan can evaluate the degree of local spread and pelvic side wall involvement. The presence of dilated or obstructed ureters or hydroneprosis suggests pelvic side wall involvement or stage III disease. A chest CT is also indicated if advanced local disease is detected to identify lung metastases. As a minimum a chest X-ray should be performed in all cases.

2. Magnetic resonance imaging (MRI). MRI is better than CT for pre-operative staging as it gives better delineation of local extent of the vaginal tumour due to its superior soft-tissue contrast. MRI has a higher sensitivity for identifying clinically occult pelvic extension into other pelvic organs such as the bladder and rectum.[9]

3. Endoscopy. Cystoscopy is rarely used, but may be helpful in cases of an equivocal pelvic MRI. Similarly, proctosigmoidoscopy may be used for unclear cases of rectal involvement. Colonoscopy should probably be performed early in the work-up of an apparent primary vaginal cancer in order to exclude a colon primary tumour. Positive findings on any of these latter tests constitute stage IV disease. Other radiological tests such as a lymphangiogram or a barium enema are rarely performed and certainly not mandatory for staging, but may help in patient management and judicious use of radiation therapy.[1]

Treatment

Several treatment options exist for patients with primary invasive carcinoma of the vagina, including radiation therapy, surgery, combination therapy with radiation and surgery and chemotherapy.[2,4–8] Although primary radiation therapy is the standard at many institutions controversy exists with regard to the best treatment regimen for patients with early stage squamous carcinomas. Recent data suggest that patients with stage I disease may have better 5-year survival outcomes when treated with surgery alone compared to radiotherapy.[2,5,7] In general, combination brachytherapy and external beam radiation is the treatment of choice for more advanced stages.[7,8] Patients with a central, non-metastatic tumour or advanced stage IV disease represent two distinct groups of patients with primary vaginal squamous carcinoma for whom a pelvic exenteration or chemotherapy may be indicated, respectively.[7]

Patients with melanomas and sarcomas represent a rare group of patients that require special consideration for treatment. Primary surgery with or without adjuvant radiotherapy is more frequently used for patients with advanced stages of melanoma. Alternatively, primary radiation may be used and is typically administered in the form of an external beam. The survival rate for patients with melanomas is poor regardless of the treatment implemented.

Women with sarcomas represent the smallest group of vaginal cancer patients. This diverse group typically has a bimodal distribution of children and women in their fifth and sixth decades. Younger patients have good long-term response rates to primary or adjuvant multi-agent chemotherapy, although primary treatment with surgery alone and radiation has also been described.[7] Older patients are more likely to undergo surgery rather than radiation or chemotherapy. In general, patient survival rates decrease with increasing age.[7]

Follow Up

Patients are reviewed 3-4 monthly for 2 years and then 6 monthly for the next 3 years. Most practitioners will undertake annual review thereafter. Review should comprise examination and vaginal vault cytology.

References

1. DeSaia PJ, Creasman WT. Invasive cancer of the vagina and urethra. In DiSaia PJ, Creasman WT (editors). *Clinical Gynecologic Oncology*, 5th edn. St Louis: C.V. Mosby; 1997: pp. 233–52.
2. Creasman WT, Phillips JL, Menck HR. The national cancer data base report on cancer of the vagina. *Cancer* 1998; **83**: 1033–40.
3. Davis KP, Stanhope CR, Garton GR *et al.* Invasive vaginal carcinoma: analysis of early-stage disease. *Gynecol Oncol* 1991; **42**: 131–6.
4. Kucera H, Vavra N. Radiation management of primary carcinoma of the vagina: clinical and histopathological variables associated with survival. *Gynecol Oncol* 1991; **40**: 12–16.
5. Tabata T, Takeshima N, Nishida H *et al.* Treatment failure in vaginal cancer. *Gynecol Oncol* 2001; **84**: 309–14.
6. Benedet JL, Bender J, Jones III H *et al.* FIGO staging classification and clinical practice guidelines in the management of gynecologic cancers. FIGO Committee on Gynecologic Oncology. *Int J Gynaecol Obstet* 2000; **70**: 209–62.
7. Tjalma WAA, Monaghan JM, Lopes ADB *et al.* The role of surgery in invasive squamous carcinoma of the vagina. *Gynecol Oncol* 2001; **81**: 360–5.
8. Tewari KS, Cappuccini F, Puthawala AA *et al.* Primary invasive carcinoma of the vagina. *Cancer* 2001; **91**: 758–70.
9. Siegelman ES, outwater EK, Banner MP *et al.* High resolution MR imaging of the vagina. *Radiographics* 1997; **17**: 1183–1203.

CARCINOMA OF THE VAGINA

† The FIGO staging system

FIGO Stage	0	I	II	III	IV	IVA	IVB
	Carcinoma *in situ* VAIN3	Carcinoma limited to the vaginal wall	Carcinoma involves subvaginal tissue, but has not extended to the pelvic wall	Carcinoma extends to the pelvic wall	Carcinoma extends beyond the true pelvis or involves mucosa of the bladder or rectum (bullous oedema does not assign a patient to stage IV)		

‡ American Joint Committee on Cancer surgical staging system

AJCC Stage	T	Tis	T1	T2	T1, 2	T3	T3		T4	any T
	N				N1	N0	N1		any N	any N
	M									M1

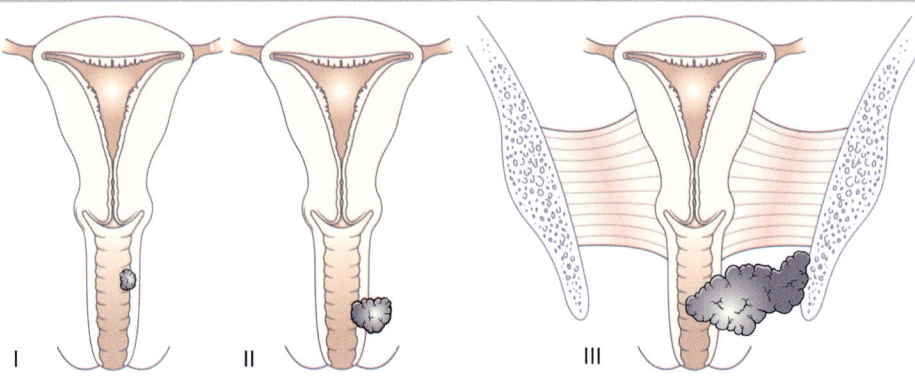
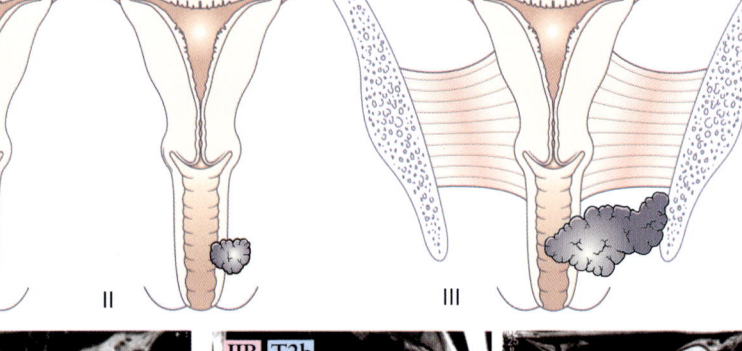
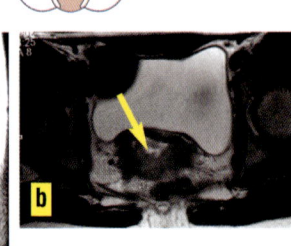
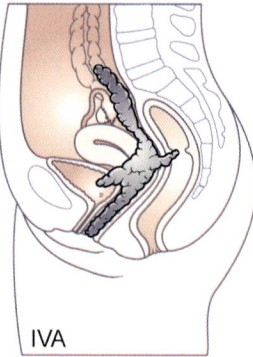

I   II   III   IVA

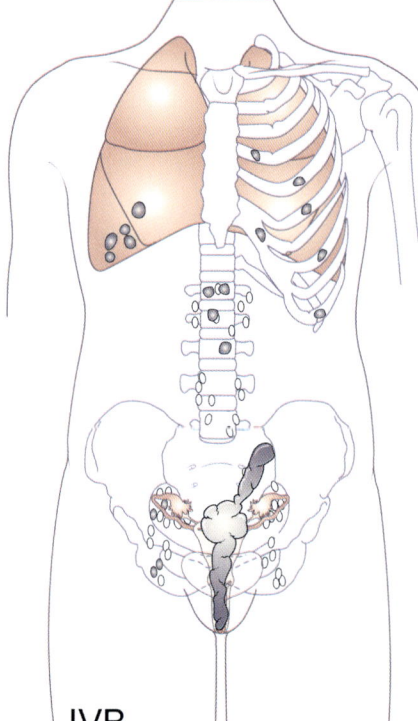

IVB

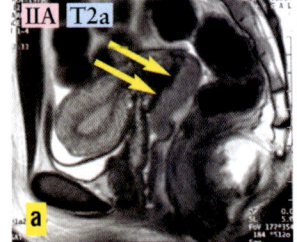
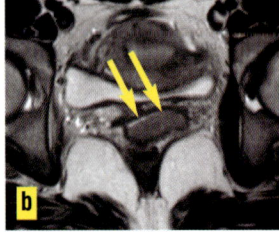

IIA T2a

T2-weighted fast-spin echo images in (a) the sagittal plane and

(b) the axial plane show a tumour (arrows) involving the posterior wall of the upper half of the vagina. The tumour is confined to the vagina.

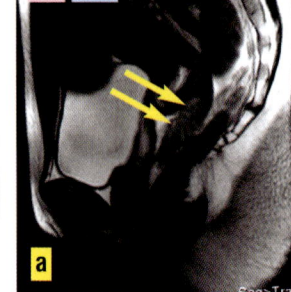

IIB T2b

T2-weighted fast-spin echo images in (a) the sagittal plane and

(b) the axial plane show a tumour (arrow) involving the posterior wall of the upper vagina with extension into the parameterium.

VULVAL CARCINOMA

S. Ghaem-Maghami, A. McIndoe, E. Moskovic and A. Sohaib

Introduction

Vulval carcinoma is predominantly a disease of post-menopausal women: in many series more than half the patients are over the age of 70 years. It accounts for approximately 3–5% of all female genital malignant neoplasms. Its incidence may be rising due to the rise in the average age in the female population.

Human papillomavirus is suspected in the aetiology of vulval cancer, but a definite causal link has not been demonstrated. Ulcerative genital disease may also be associated with vulval neoplasia.

The most common histological type is squamous cell carcinoma, accounting for 90% of cases, followed by malignant melanoma; other rarer histological types also occur.

Vulval intraepithelial neoplasia (VIN), which occurs in younger women, is regarded as a pre-cancerous state for vulval carcinoma. After histological diagnosis careful consideration should be given to the management of VIN III usually either by excision, laser therapy or careful observation.

As vulval carcinoma is a relatively rare condition, it is best managed in cancer centres where relevant expertise exists to provide individualized multidisciplinary care for patients with this condition.

Staging

In order to manage vulval cancer optimally the disease should be staged accurately and histological assessment of the lesion carried out. The current predominantly surgical staging of vulval carcinoma was introduced in 1988. Final staging is made after examination of the surgical specimen from the vulva and the lymph nodes (if these are removed).

Malignant melanomas are staged according to the system for cutaneous melanomas and should be recorded separately.

ANATOMY AND SPREAD

Cases are classified as carcinoma of the vulva only if the primary site of growth is in the vulva. Secondary deposits on the vulva from other malignancies should be excluded. The inguinal and femoral nodes are the primary sites of regional spread. If pelvic lymph nodes become involved with disease, these are regarded as distant metastases.

Regional lymph nodes (N)

NX: regional lymph nodes cannot be assessed.

NO: no regional lymph node metastasis.

N1: unilateral regional lymph node metastasis.

N2: bilateral regional lymph node metastasis.

Distant metastasis (M)

MX: distant metastasis cannot be assessed.

M0: no distant metastasis.

M1: distant metastasis.

Histopathological types/grades

The main histopathological types are as follows.

Squamous cell carcinoma.

Malignant melanoma.

Adenocarcinoma underlying Paget's disease of the vulva.

Verrucous carcinoma.

Bartholin's gland carcinoma.

Adenocarcinoma not otherwise specified.

Basal cell carcinoma can also occur in the vulva.

Histopathological grades (G) are divided into four categories.

Gx: grade cannot be assessed.
G1: well differentiated.
G2: moderately differentiated.
G3: poorly differentiated

International Federation of Gynecology and Obstetrics staging

The anatomical staging system for vulval carcinoma[1] of the International Federation of Gynecology and Obstetrics (Federation Internationale Gynecologique Obstetrique or FIGO) describes stage 0 as carcinoma *in situ* (pre-invasive carcinoma or VIN3).

Stage I is when a tumour measuring 2 cm or less in its greatest dimension is confined to the vulva or vulva and perineum. Stage II is defined as a tumour that measures more than 2 cm confined to the vulva or vulva and perineum and in stage III the tumour involves the lower urethra, vagina, anus or unilateral groin nodes. The FIGO classification, which was introduced in 1988 for vulval carcinoma, reclassified bilateral groin node involvement as stage IVa, while involvement of the bladder, rectum or upper urethral mucosa also fall into this category. Any distant metastasis, including pelvic nodes (external, hypogastric, obturator or common iliac), is classified as stage IVB.

If the general staging system of the International Union Against Cancer (UICC) classification of cancer is used, that is the TNM (tumour, node, metastasis) classification, carcinoma of vulva can be categorized as seen in the atlas spread on pages 12 and 13.

Principal Investigations

Principal investigations for patients with vulval carcinoma

1. Colposcopy of the cervix and vagina and cervical cytology because of the common association with other squamous intraepithelial lesions.

2. Computed tomography (CT) scanning. CT scan of the pelvis can detect enlarged lymph nodes but has a low sensitivity for detecting malignant lymphadenopathy. CT of the chest and abdomen can detect distant metastatic disease.

3. Ultrasound can be a useful tool for evaluating lymph nodes but is highly operator dependent. Ultrasound benefits from the ability to guide fine needle aspiration for cytological analysis of suspicious groin nodes.

4. Magnetic resonance imaging (MRI) may be used in place of CT for the assessment of groin and pelvic lymph nodes.

5. Sentinel node mapping may have an increasing role, but its precise clinical utility is yet to be defined – despite this the results of the sentinel node assessment can be used in staging and determining surgical effort.

6. A full blood count and biochemical profile are normally checked prior to surgery.

Treatment

TREATMENT OF VULVAL LESIONS
Micro-invasive vulval cancer
Micro-invasive vulval cancer, which is defined as a single lesion measuring less than 2 cm in maximum diameter and with a depth of invasion less than or equal to 1.0 mm, is usually managed by complete local excision of the lesion only.

Invasive vulval cancer
No clinical evidence of lymphadenopathy
In stage I and II lesions with no clinical evidence of lymph node enlargement, a wedge biopsy is performed in order to assess the depth of invasion and rule out the presence of micro-invasive disease. If the depth of invasion is confirmed to be more than 1 mm then a radical local excision and unilateral inguinofemoral node dissection is the treatment of choice. Bilateral nodal dissection is indicated if the lesion is situated in the midline, if the labia minora are involved or there are positive ipsilateral lymph nodes. This is based on the observation that, in early lateral tumours, the incidence of positive contra-lateral nodes is less than 1%.[2]

Surgical removal should achieve lateral margins of at least 1 cm and deep margins should be to the inferior fascia of the urogenital diaphragm and the fascia over the symphysis pubis. If the lesion is close to the urethra, the lower 1 cm of the urethra may be removed with a low possibility of causing urinary incontinence. If histologically the surgical margins are less than 5 mm careful consideration should be given to radiotherapy.

In certain cases of locally advanced tumours, if the tumour does not appear to be resectable without requiring a stoma, pre-operative radiotherapy and chemotherapy should be considered prior to resection of the tumour bed.

Groin node dissection
A triple incision may be used safely and carries less morbidity than an *en bloc* approach. It is recommended that both the inguinal and femoral nodes be removed as resecting the inguinal node alone is associated with a higher incidence of groin recurrence.[3] If there is more than one (or possibly two) nodal metastasis of less than 5 mm no adjuvant therapy is indicated. However, the patient should receive pelvic irradiation if there is one or more macro-metastases (larger than 10 mm), if there is extra-capsular spread or if there are two (or possibly three) or more micro-metastases.

Clinical evidence of lymphadenopathy
If the groin nodes are grossly enlarged and either fixed or ulcerated, histological confirmation of the diagnosis is advisable. Surgical excision should be considered for all macroscopic enlarged nodes in the groin and enlarged nodes seen on CT prior to radiotherapy. A full inguinofemoral lymphadenectomy should be avoided in order to avoid severe lymphoedema. If the nodes are deemed not resectable, pre-operative radiotherapy with or without chemotherapy is advised. This should then be followed by post-operative resection of macroscopic residual disease.

Follow Up
Patients are reviewed 3-4 monthly for 2 years and then 6 monthly for the next 3 years. Most practitioners will undertake annual review thereafter. Review should comprise examination only and not vulval cytology.

References

1. Benedet MD, Pecorelli S. Staging classifications and clinical practice guidelines of gynaecologic cancers. FIGO Committee on Gynaecologic Oncology. *Int J Gynecol Obstet* 2000; **70:** 207–312.
2. Hacker NF. Vulval cancer. In Berek JS, Hacker NF (editors). *Practical Gynaecologic Oncology,* 3rd edn. Williams and Wilkins; 1994, 2000.
3. Stehman FB, Bundy BN, Doretsky PM, Creasman WT. Early stage I carcinoma of the vulva treated with ipsilateral superficial inguinal lymphadenectomy and modified radical hemi-vulvectomy: a prospective study of the Gynaecologic Oncology Group. *Obstet Gynecol* 1992; **79:** 490.
4. Sohaib SA, Richards PS, Ind T *et al.* MR imaging of carcinoma of the vulva. *Am J Roentgenol* 2002; **178**(2): 373–7.

† The FIGO staging system

FIGO Stage	Primary tumour cannot be assessed	No evidence of primary tumour	**0** Carcinoma in situ (pre-invasive carcinoma) (VIN 3)	**I** Tumour confined to the vulva or vulva and perineum, 2 cm or less in greatest dimension	**IA** Tumour confined to the vulva or vulva and perineum, 2 cm or less in greatest dimension with stromal invasion no greater than 1.0 mm	**IB** Tumour confined to the vulva or vulva and perineum, 2 cm or less in greatest dimension with stromal invasion greater than 1.0 mm	**II** Tumour confined to the vulva or vulva and perineum, more than 2 cm in greatest dimension

‡ American Joint Committee on Cancer surgical staging system

AJCC Stage	T	**TX**	**T0**	**Tis**	**T1**	**T1a**	**T1b**	**T2**
	N							
	M							

T F N
The depth of invasion is measured from the epithelial–stromal junction of the adjacent-most superficial normal dermal papilla to the deepest point of cancer invasion.

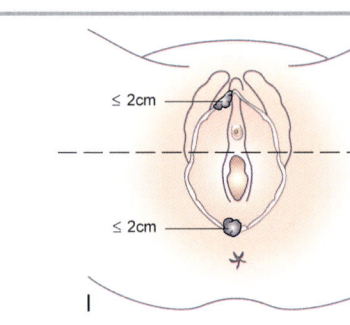

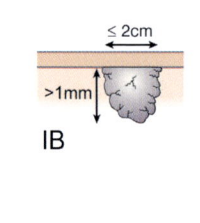

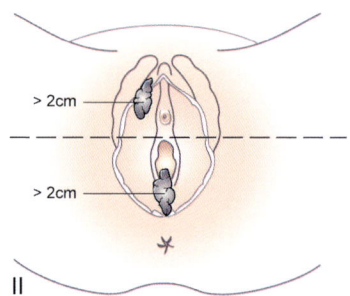

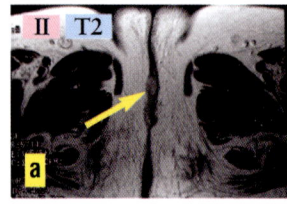
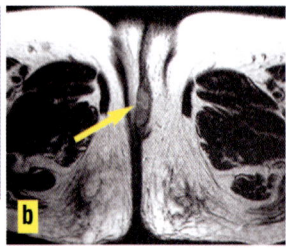

Vulval carcinoma. (a) and (b) Axial T2-weighted fast-spin echo images show a tumour (arrows) of 3 cm involving the left labia.

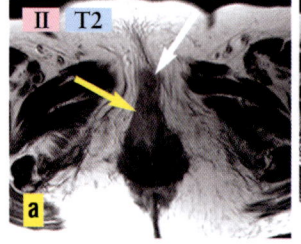
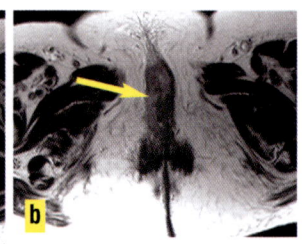

Vulval carcinoma involving the clitoris. (a) and (b) Axial T2-weighted fast-spin echo images show a tumour (yellow arrow) involving the right labia and extending to involve the clitoris (white arrow).

III

Tumour invades any of the following: the lower urethra, vagina, anus and/or unilateral regional node metastasis

IVA

Tumour invades any of the following: the bladder mucosa, rectal mucosa or upper urethral mucosa or is fixed to bone and/or bilateral regional node metastasis

IVB

Any distant metastasis including pelvic nodes

**T1, 2, 3
N1**

**T1, 2, 3
N2**   **T4
any N**

**any T
any N
M1**

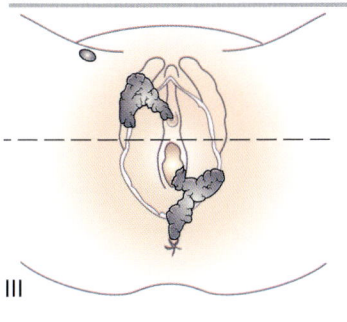
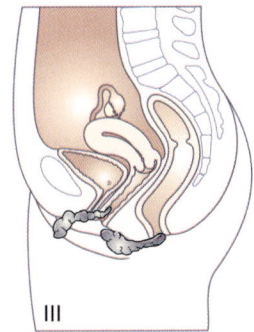

III

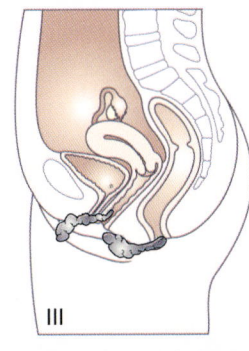

III

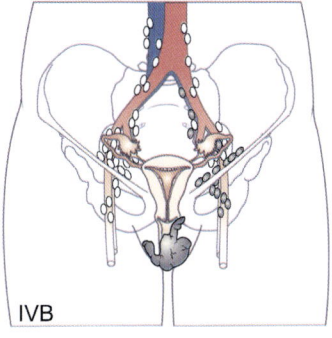

IVB

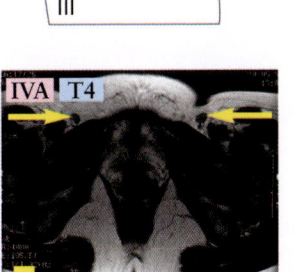

Vulval carcinoma. (a) and (b) Axial T2-weighted fast-spin echo images show an involved left inguinal lymph node (arrow). The primary lesion, which was 3 cm in maximum length but only 1 mm deep, could not be seen on MRI.

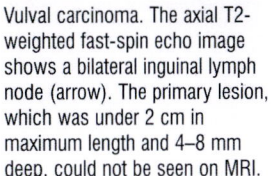

Vulval carcinoma. The axial T2-weighted fast-spin echo image shows a bilateral inguinal lymph node (arrow). The primary lesion, which was under 2 cm in maximum length and 4–8 mm deep, could not be seen on MRI.

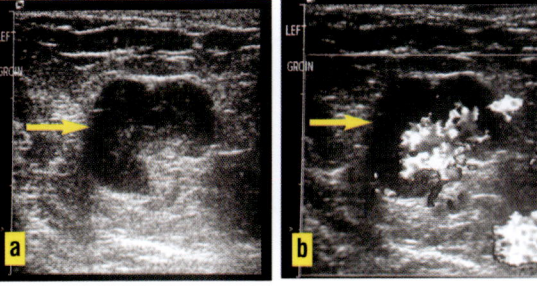
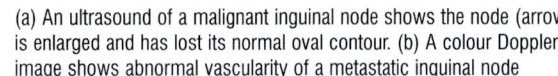

(a) An ultrasound of a malignant inguinal node shows the node (arrow) is enlarged and has lost its normal oval contour. (b) A colour Doppler image shows abnormal vascularity of a metastatic inguinal node

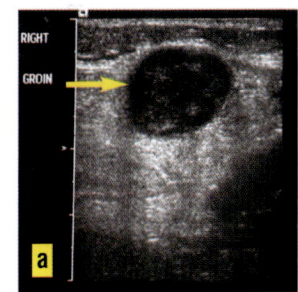

An ultrasound of a malignant inguinal node shows the node (arrow) is large and circular in contour with loss of normal sinus/hilar echogenicity

ENDOMETRIAL CANCER

A. Wang, K.M. Hartzfeld and M. Hughes

Introduction

Endometrial cancer is the most common gynaecological malignancy in the USA, accounting for 6% of all new cancer diagnoses in women. The prognosis is relatively good, since most cases (73%) are diagnosed at an early stage when surgery alone is sufficient for cure. The 5-year survival rates for localized, regional and metastatic disease are 96, 65 and 26%, respectively.[1]

Staging

Surgical staging

According to the revised classification system of the International Federation of Gynecology and Obstetrics (Federation Internationale Gynecologique Obstetrique or FIGO) endometrial cancer is surgically staged by means of a total abdominal hysterectomy with bilateral salpingo-oophorectomy (TAH-BSO) and lymph node sampling from the pelvis and para-aortic areas. In addition, peritoneal washings and a complete examination of the abdominal contents should be performed. The stage should be assigned at the time of definitive surgical exploration and treatment, prior to radiation or chemotherapy. The depth of myometrial invasion should be noted intra-operatively as well as on the final pathology report. The final pathology report may also contain a description of the myometrial thickness and distance from the serosa at that portion of the uterine wall representing the deepest invasion.[2]

The presence of carcinoma in regional lymph nodes may be of critical prognostic value and lymph node sampling is mandated for the current staging system. However, according to FIGO treatment guidelines, this procedure may be omitted in cases where tumour involvement is limited to the endometrium. Surgical staging may also be limited by the presence of co-morbid conditions such as extreme obesity or life threatening heart disease when the risk of lymph node involvement is low. After lymphatic spread, metastases are typically either direct or hematogeneous, with spread extending from the pelvic and para-aortic nodes to the lung, inguinal and supraclavicular nodes, liver, lung, peritoneal cavity, bone, brain and vagina.

The surgical stages set by FIGO correspond to the definitions of the TNM (tumour, node, metastasis) categories established by the American Joint Committee on Cancer (AJCC)[3].

Clinical staging

Clinical staging may be performed in selected cases where surgical staging presents an unacceptable risk. Guidelines for clinical staging were set by FIGO in 1971.[2] The greater accuracy of surgical staging is clearly demonstrated in one large study of 6085 women. The study compared survival of patients with the previously used clinical staging to those with surgical staging. Clinical stage I disease, was comparable to that of surgical stage III disease. Those clinically at stage III were similar to patients with surgical stage IV disease.[4] Thus, the more accurate surgical staging recommended by the AJCC and FIGO should be performed whenever possible. Adjuvant treatment can then be prescribed on the basis of the staging information.

Histopathologic grade

Cases are grouped according to the degree of differentiation of the adenocarcinoma as follows.[2]

G1: 5% or less of a non-squamous or non-morular solid growth pattern.

G2: 6–50% of a non-squamous or non-morular solid growth pattern.

G3: greater than 50% of a non-squamous or non-morular solid growth pattern.

Notable nuclear atypia, out of proportion to the architectural grade, raises the grade to G3.

Principal Investigations

Endometrial biopsy

The largest study of the prognostic value of endometrial sampling involved a meta-analysis of 39 studies involving 7914 women. The results of endometrial sampling were compared to more invasive techniques, such as dilatation and curettage, hysteroscopy and hysterectomy. The detection rates for endometrial cancer were 99.6% in post-menopausal women and 91% for pre-menopausal women. The overall detection rate for atypical hyperplasia was 81%. The specificity for all sampling types was in the range 98–100%. An insufficient sample was returned in as many as 5% of patients.[5] Therefore, endometrial biopsy might be an appropriate initial diagnostic test for ruling out endometrial cancer in symptomatic women. More invasive diagnostic methods may be considered in cases where the sample was inadequate. The overall grade for the patient's tumour is based on the worse sample obtained, whether from the biopsy, dilatation and curettage or hysterectomy specimen.

Ultrasound

Transvaginal ultrasound is another accurate method of evaluating the endometrium of symptomatic patients. To perform this study, a view of the uterus is obtained in the sagittal view. The double wall thickness of the endometrium is then measured in an anteroposterior dimension from one basalis layer to the other. Any fluid within the cavity should be excluded from measurement.[6] Using this method, an endometrial thickness of less than 5 mm is associated with a low but not negligible risk of endometrial disease.[7] A thicker lining warrants further evaluation in at-risk patients.

A large meta-analysis of almost 6000 women supported this finding. In this study, the post-test probability of cancer was less than 1% for an asymptomatic post-menopausal woman with an endometrial thickness of less than 5 mm. However, other studies have found that the detection rate for endometrial cancer varies according to the cut-off for abnormality and noted that the median endometrial thickness varies between centres.[8] Another large meta-analysis evaluated 9031 patients. Four studies used the cut-off of 5 mm. A positive test raised the probability of carcinoma from a pre-test 14% to a post-test 31%, while a negative test reduced it to 2.5%. The authors concluded that the ultrasound measurement could not be used alone to rule out endometrial cancer.

The depth of invasion, size and location of the tumour are also important prognostic factors obtained from ultrasound. They are not used for official staging, but can guide decisions on treatment or the planned surgery. For instance, larger tumours, i.e. >2 cm, deeper invasion, i.e. >30% and lower uterine segment involvement are all associated with an increase risk of metastatic disease.

Computed tomography scanning

Computed tomography (CT) scanning is rarely necessary, except in cases where there is evidence of extensive disease. Therefore, it may be indicated when there is evidence of extra-pelvic spread on physical examination, symptoms or pre-operative high-risk factors. A pre-operative endometrial biopsy indicating papillary serous, carcinoma, sarcoma or other high-risk histology may also indicate a potential benefit for a pre-operative CT of the pelvis, abdomen and chest. However, in general, several studies have shown that CT scans would not alter treatment and have only low sensitivity for myometrial invasion, cervical extension and nodal involvement.[9–11] It is also not used for the official staging assignment.

Magnetic resonance imaging

Contrast-enhanced magnetic resonance imaging (MRI) appears to be the best radiographic modality for assessing myometrial invasion and tumour size and location. It appears to be significantly more sensitive than ultrasound, CT and non-enhanced MRI[12] and correlates well with gross visual inspection.[13] A meta-analysis of studies using MRI for diagnosing the presence of myometrial invasion (1875 patients) obtained a positive likelihood ratio of 10.11 and a negative likelihood ratio of 0.1.[14] One small study (25 patients) suggested that MRI may have a similar cost and accuracy to intra-operative surgical and pathologic staging and may decrease the number of lymph node dissections.[15] Like CT, lymph node status is based on the arbitrary size cut-off used, typically 1 cm, for determining a 'positive' node. As a result, the sensitivity and specificity vary inversely: smaller size cut-offs increase the sensitivity, but at the expense of a decrease in specificity.

Although promising, these results are preliminary and MRI has not been established as a replacement for surgical lymph node dissection for official purposes.

Serum CA125

Measurement of pre-operative CA125 may prove to be useful in predicting the extra-uterine spread of endometrial cancer. Some studies have shown a correlation between CA125 levels and the extent of disease.[16–18] However, the optimal cut-off level has not been established and a normal level cannot be considered sufficient justification for the avoidance of surgical staging.

Management

Treatment recommendations depend on the estimated risk of recurrent disease, which is based upon surgical stage, tumour grade and histological subtype. These general management guidelines apply to the most common type, endometrioid adenocarcinoma.

Low risk

Patients with endometrial cancer must meet the following criteria to be considered low-risk patients.[19]

- Grade 1–2 histology, with invasion through less than 33% of the myometrium.
- Grade 3 without myometrial invasion.
- Disease confined to the uterine fundus.
- No lymphovascular involvement.
- No evidence of metastases.

TAH-BSO is the definitive treatment in these cases. The prognosis is good: one study of 670 patients showed that patients treated with surgery had a 5-year survival rate of 98%, with 93% disease free. Recurrence is less than 7% and can be successfully salvaged with radiotherapy.[20] For patients who present a significant surgical risk, primary radiotherapy may be considered. The 5-year survival rates in one study of 171 patients were 76% and 71% for stages IA and IB, respectively.[21]

Intermediate risk

Patients are considered at intermediate risk if they have the following.

- Grade 1–2 histology with more than 50% invasion of the myometrium.
- Invasion of the cervix or isthmus.
- No involvement of the lymphovascular space.
- No evidence of metastases.

The discrepancy between 33% and 50%

depth of myometrial invasion reflects different study definitions. Depth of invasion is a continuous variable which is arbitrarily divided into categories with no physiological correlate. These women should receive a TAH-BSO with lymphadenectomy. Traditionally, vaginal or pelvic adjuvant radiotherapy was often recommended for these patients.[22] However, a recent study of 448 patients found the projected 4-year survival rate was not significantly different although there was a lower 2-year cumulative incidence of recurrence in patients receiving adjunctive external beam radiation.[23]

High risk

Patients with any of the following characteristics are considered high risk.

- Grade 3 histology with any degree of myometrial invasion.
- Adnexal or pelvic metastases.
- Grade 2 disease with invasion greater than 50% of the myometrium and uterine extension beyond the fundus.
- Involvement of the lymphovascular spaces.

The prognosis of women with high-risk disease with surgery alone is poor. Some studies have suggested the benefit of surgical cytoreduction in stage IV disease.[24–26] The optimal modality of adjuvant therapy is controversial. There is some evidence that radiation therapy (including vaginal cuff brachytherapy, pelvic external beam radiation and whole abdominal irradiation) reduces local recurrence and may prolong survival.[27] There may also be a benefit in 5-year disease-free survival rates when cisplatin, doxorubicin and cyclophosphamide are used.[28] An unpublished randomized trial from the GOG comparing radiation and chemotherapy indicates that chemotherapy may be best for adjuvant therapy in advanced disease.

Follow-up

Recurrent endometrial cancer usually manifests within the first 3 years after diagnosis and treatment: estimates vary from 75 to 95%.[19] The signs and symptoms suggestive of recurrent disease include bleeding (vaginal, rectal or bladder), pelvic pain, cough, dyspnoea, anorexia or unexplained weight loss. According to the National Comprehensive Cancer Network post-operative surveillance should consist of the following.[29]

- A physical examination every 3–6 months for 2 years.

- A physical examination every 6 months to 1 year after 2 years.

- Vaginal cytology every 6 months for 2 years, then annually. (This is usually omitted in the UK but speculum and vaginal examination should take place).

- An annual chest X-ray. (This is often omitted in the UK).

This surveillance programme rarely detects aysmptomatic recurrences, but it continues to be widely employed.

References

1. Jemal A, Tiwari RC, Murray T et al. Cancer statistics, 2004. Cancer 2004; 54(1): 8-29.
2. Benedet JL, Bender H, Jones III H et al. Staging classifications and clinical practice guidelines in the management of gynaecologic cancers. FIGO Committee on Gynecologic Oncology. Int J Gyaecol Obstetr 2000 Aug; 70(2): 209-62.
3. American Joint Committee on Cancer. In: Greene FL, Balch CM, Page DL et al. (editors). Cancer Staging Manual, 6th edn. Chicago: Springer; 2002.
4. Creasman W, Odicino F, Maisonneuve P et al. Carcinoma of the corpus uteri: FIGO annual report. J Epidemiol Biostat 2001; 6(1): 47-86.
5. Dijkhuizen FP, Mol BW, Brolmann HA, Heintz AP. The accuracy of endometrial sampling in the diagnosis of patients with endometrial carcinoma and hyperplasia: a meta-analysis. Cancer 2000 Oct 15; 89(8): 1765-72.
6. Goldstein RB, Bree RL, Benson CB et al. Evaluation of the woman with postmenopausal bleeding: Society of Radiologists in Ultrasound - sponsored Consensus Conference Statement. J Ultrasound Med. 2001 Oct; 20(10): 1025-36.
7. Goldstein SR, Nachticall M, Snyder JR et al. Endometrial assessment by vaginal ultrasonography before endometrial sampling in patients with postmenopausal bleeding. Am J Obstet Gynecol 1990 Jul; 163(1 Pt 1): 119-23.
8. Tabor A, Watt HC, Wald NJ. Endometrial thickness as a test for endometrial cancer in women with postmenopausal vaginal bleeding. Obstet Gynecol 2002 Apr; 99(4): 663-70.
9. Connor JO, Andrews JI, Anderson B et al. Computed tomography in endometrial cancer. Obstet Gynecol 2000 May; 95(5): 692-6.
10. Zerbe MJ, Bristow R, Grumbine FC et al. Inability of preoperative computed tomography scans to accurately predict the extent of myometrial invasion and extracorporeal spread in endometrial cancer. Gynecol Oncol 2000 Jul; 78(1): 67-70.
11. Hardesty LA, Sumkin JH, Hakim C et al. The ability of helical CT to preoperatively stage endometrial carcinoma. Am J Radiol 2001 Mar; 176(3): 603-6.
12. Kinkel K, Kahi Y, Yu KK et al. Radiologic staging in patients with endometrial cancer: a meta-analysis. Radiology 1999 Sep; 212(3): 711-8.
13. Cunha TM, Felix A, Cabral J. Preoperative assessment of deep myometrial and cervical invasion in endometrial carcinoma: comparison of magnetic resonance imaging and gross visual inspection. Int J Gynecol Cancer 2001 Mar-Apr; 11(2): 130-6.
14. Frei KA, Kinkel K, Bonel HM et al. Prediction of deep myometrial invasion in patients with endometrial cancer: clinical utility of contrast-enhanced MR imaging – a meta-analysis and Bayesian analysis. Radiology 2000 Aug; 216(2): 444-9.
15. Hardesty LA, Sumkin JH, Nath ME et al. Use of preoperative MR imaging in the management of endometrial carcinoma: cost analysis. Radiology 2000 Apr; 215(1): 45-9.
16. Hsieh CH, Chang-Chien CC, Lin H et al. Can a preoperative CA125 level be a criterion for full pelvic lymphadenectomy in surgical staging of endometrial cancer? Gynecol Oncol 2002 Jul; 86(1): 28-33.
17. Ebina Y, Sakuragi N, Hareyama H et al. Para-aortic lymph node metastasis in relation to serum CA125 levels and nuclear grade in endometrial carcinoma. Acta Obstet Gynecol Stand 2002 May; 81(5): 458–65.
18. Dotters DJ. Preoperative CA125 in endometrial cancer: is it useful? Am J Obstet Gynecol 2000 Jun; 182(6): 1328-34.
19. Morrow CP, Bundy BN, Kurman RJ et al. Relationship between surgical–pathological risk factors and outcome in clinical stage I and II carcinoma of the endometrium: a Gynecologic Oncology Group study. Gynecol Oncol 1991 Jan; 40(1): 55-65.
20. Straughn JM, Huh WK, Kelly FJ et al. Conservative management of stage I endometrial carcinoma after surgical staging. Gynecol Oncol 2002 Feb; 84(2): 194-200.
21. Lehoczky L, Bosze P, Ungar L et al. Stage I endometrial carcinoma: treatment of nonoperable patients with intracavitary radiation therapy alone. Gynecol Oncol 1991 Dec; 43(3): 211-6.
22. Nag S, Erickson B, Parikh S et al. The American Brachytherapy Society recommendations for high-dose-rate brachytherapy for carcinoma of the endometrium. Int J Radiat Oncol Biol Phys 2000; 48(3): 779-90.
23. Keys HM, Roberts JA, Brunetto VL et al. A phase III trial of surgery with or without adjunctive external pelvic radiation therapy in intermediate risk endometrial adenocarcinoma: a Gynecologic Oncology Group study. Gynecol Oncol 2004 Mar; 92(3): 744-51.
24. Chi DS, Welshinger M, Venkatraman ES et al. The role of surgical cytoreduction in stage IV endometrial cancer. Gynecol Oncol 1997 Oct; 67(1): 56-60.
25. Bristow RE, Zerbe MJ, Rosenshein NB et al. Stage IVB endometrial carcinoma: the role of cytoreductive surgery and determinants of survival. Gynecol Oncol 2000 Aug; 78(2): 85-91.
26. Ayhan A, Taskiran C, Celik C et al. The influence of cytoreductive surgery on survival and morbidity in stage IVB endometrial cancer. Int J Gynecol Cancer 2002 Sep-Oct; 12(5): 448-53.
27. Grigsby PW. Update on radiation therapy for endometrial cancer. Oncology 2002 Jun; 16(6): 777-86, 790.
28. Aoki Y, Kase H, Watanabe M et al. Stage III endometrial cancer: analysis of prognostic factors and failure patterns after adjuvant chemotherapy. Gynecol Oncol 2001 Oct; 83(1): 1-5.
29. Teng N, Abu-Rustum N, Bookman M et al. Practice Guidelines in Oncology: Uterine Cancers – v.1.2003. National Comprehensive Cancer Network; 2004.

CARCINOMA OF THE CORPUS UTERI

FIGO Stage	Primary tumour cannot be assessed	No evidence of primary tumour	**0** Carcinoma in situ (pre-invasive carcinoma)	**I** Tumour confined to the corpus uteri	**IA** Tumour limited to the endometrium	**IB** Tumour invades up to less than half of the myometrium	**IC** Tumour invades to more than one half of the myometrium	**II** Tumour invades the cervix but does not extend beyond the uterus	**IIA** Endocervical glandular involvement only

AJCC Stage	T	TX	T0	Tis	T1	T1a	T1b	T1c	T2	T2a
	N									
	M									

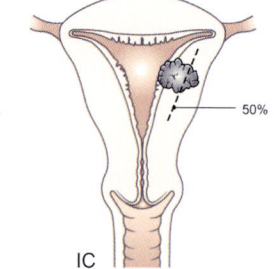
IA   IB   IC
50%   50%

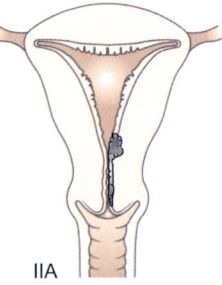
IIA
Tumour extending into the cervical canal without invasion of the cervical stroma

Normal myometrium

intact uterine junctional zone

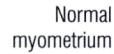 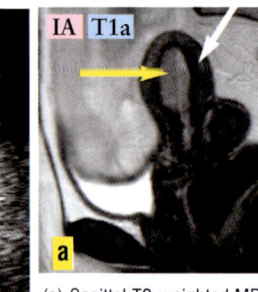
IA **T1a**

Transverse ultrasound section through the uterine body showing the endometrial cavity expanded by an echogenic endometrial carcinoma. The tumour is confined to the endometrial cavity with no extension into the myometrium.

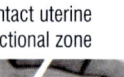 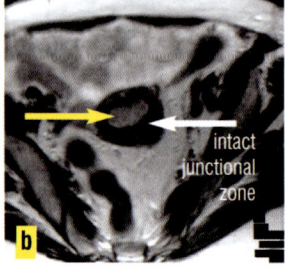
IA **T1a**

a

(a) Sagittal T2-weighted MRI through the uterus showing a high-signal tumour confined to the endometrial cavity. There is no extension of the carcinoma through the surrounding low signal myometrial junctional zone.

b

intact junctional zone

(b) Axial T2-weighted MRI through the body of the uterus in the same patient as (a) showing the high-signal endometrial carcinoma confined to the endometrial cavity and surrounded by an intact junctional zone.

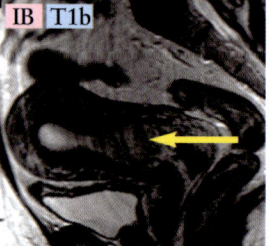
IB **T1b**

Sagittal T2-weighted MRI showing an intermediate-signal endometrial carcinoma extending through the junctional zone, but invading less than one-half of the myometrium.

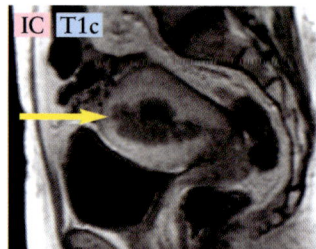
IC **T1c**

Sagittal T2-weighted MRI showing an intermediate signal endometrial carcinoma extending through the junctional zone, but invading less than one-half of the myometrium.

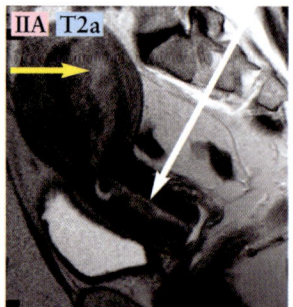
IIA **T2a**

Sagittal T2-weighted MRI showing an endometrial carcinoma extending into the cervical canal, but not invading the cervical stroma. The carcinoma within the body of the uterus has breached the junctional zone posteriorly.

IIB	**III**	**IIIA**	**IIIB**	**IIIC**	**IVA**	**IVB**
Cervical stromal invasion	Local and/or regional spread as specified in stages IIIA, B and C	Tumour involves the serosa and/or adnexa (direct extension or metastasis) and/or cancer cells in ascites or peritoneal washings	Vaginal involvement (direct extension or metastasis)	Metastasis to the pelvic and/or para-aortic lymph nodes	Tumour invades the bladder mucosa and/or bowel mucosa	Distant metastasis (excluding metastasis to the vagina, pelvic serosa or adnexa, including metastasis to intra-abdominal lymph nodes other than para-aortic and/or inguinal nodes)
T2b	**T3** **and/or N1**	**T3a**	**T3b**	**T1, 2, 3, 3a, 3b** **N1**	**T4** **any N**	**any T** **any N** **M1**

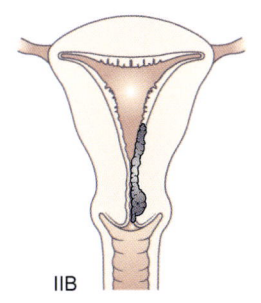

IIB

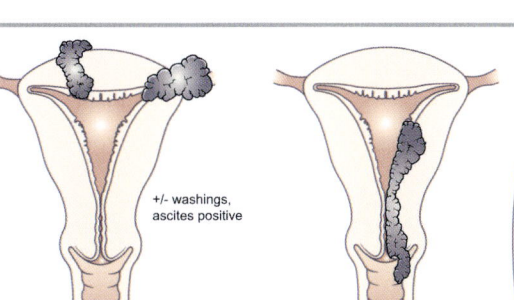

IIIA

+/- washings, ascites positive

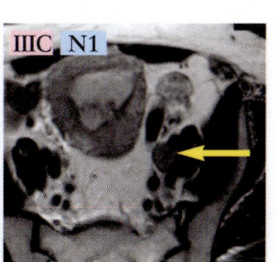

IIIB

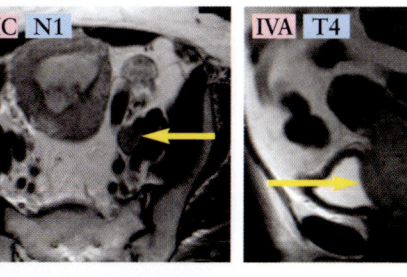

IIIC

IVA

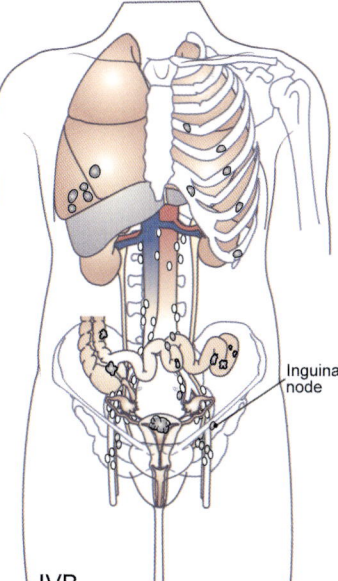

Inguinal node

IVB

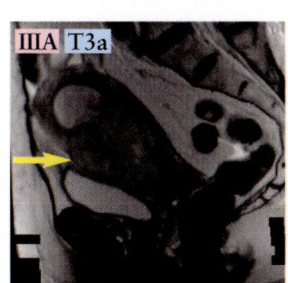

IIB T2b

Sagittal T2-weighted MRI showing an endometrial carcinoma extending into the cervical canal and invading the cervical stroma. The tumour is confined by the junctional zone within the body of the uterus.

IIIA T3a

Sagittal T2-weighted MRI demonstrating an endometrial carcinoma invading the uterine serosa anteriorly. The tumour is contacting but not invading the bladder wall.

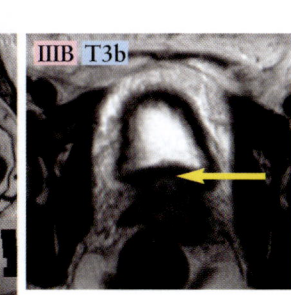

IIIB T3b

Axial T2-weighted MRI at the level of the cervico–vaginal junction showing an intermediate-signal endometrial carcinoma extending into the vagina.

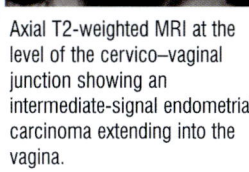

IIIC N1

Endometrial carcinoma FIGO stage IIIC/TNM stage N1. Axial T2-weighted MRI through the body of the cervix demonstrating an enlarged left obturator lymph node in keeping with metastatic involvement. The endometrial cavity is distended by the primary endometrial carcinoma.

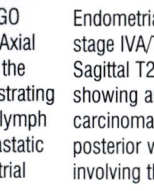

IVA T4

Endometrial carcinoma FIGO stage IVA/TNM stage T4. Sagittal T2-weighted MRI showing an endometrial carcinoma invading through the posterior wall of the bladder and involving the bladder epithelium.

19

OVARIAN CANCER

S. Shahabi and A. Sohaib

Introduction

Ovarian cancer constitutes nearly 4% of all cancers among women and is the leading cause of death from gynaecological malignancies in the Western world. It was estimated that 24 400 new cases of ovarian cancer would be diagnosed and 14 300 deaths would occur from ovarian cancer in the USA in 2003. The overall incidence rate in the USA is 17.1 per 100 000 women and has been fairly stable over time.[1] The age-specific incidence of ovarian cancer increases with age and peaks in the eighth decade. The median age of diagnosis is 63 years. Tumours of the ovary form a heterogeneous group of neoplasms. The surface epithelium, stroma and germ cells each cause an array of histogenetically distinctive tumours that can occur in pure or combined forms.[2] Malignant epithelial tumours account for approximately 85% of ovarian cancers. Age at diagnosis, race, stage of the disease, tumour grade and histological type of tumour have all been shown to have a significant impact on prognosis. An improved relative survival of women with primary epithelial ovarian cancer over the past three decades has been reported.[1]

Staging

A cancer staging system must reflect the biological behaviour of the cancer by dividing the patients into prognostic subgroups based on disease extent and other factors. Staging also facilitates treatment planning and the comparison of data between institutions.

The International Federation of Gynecology and Obstetrics (Federation Internationale Gynecologique Obstetrique or FIGO) system is the most commonly used staging system. It is based on the current understanding of the major patterns of disease spread: direct extension, exfoliation and lymphatic dissemination.[2] The extent of the tumour spread is determined by a systematic surgical procedure.[3] Stage I is tumour confined to the ovaries, stage II includes peritoneal metastasis within the true pelvis, stage III consists of abdominal peritoneal implants or retroperitoneal lymphadenopathy and stage IV involves other sites or the liver parenchyma. An alternative staging system is the American Joint Committee on Cancer (AJCC) TNM (tumour, node, metastasis) classification.

Principal Investigations

Biomarker level determinations

The serum levels of CA125 generally reflect the volume of the disease. Elevated CA125 prior to surgery is useful for following the progress of the patient during and after treatment. CA15-3, CA19-9 and lipophosphatidic acid have been shown to have independent expression to CA125. Lactate dehydrogenase, human chorionic gonadotrophin and Alfa Feto Protein are used in the diagnosis of different types of germ cell tumours. Inhibin is performed only in post-menopausal women with granulose cell tumours.[4]

Transvaginal ultrasound with Doppler studies

This is the modality of choice in the evaluation of patients with suspected adnexal masses. Combined morphological and vascular imaging obtained by transvaginal ultrasound will improve the pre-operative assessment of adnexal masses. Three-dimensional sonography and power Doppler imaging has been shown to be a better tool for assessing suspected ovarian lesions.[5]

Pathology

Cytological analysis of ascites and pleural effusions should be performed prior to a therapeutic decision. While biopsy of an isolated ovarian mass is rarely indicated, a fine-needle aspirate or biopsy specimen of a metastatic lesion is commonly useful.

Computed tomography scanning

This is currently the primary imaging modality for diagnosis and follow-up of the extent of the disease. Computed tomography (CT) scanning can identify peritoneal metastases down to the size of approximately 5 mm. The advent of thin section, spiral and now multislice CT has improved its overall accuracy in staging.

Magnetic resonance imaging scanning (MRI)

This modality seems to be a more accurate way of detecting peritoneal metastases outside the true pelvis.[6]

Combined fluoro-2-deoxyglucose–positron emission tomography (PET-CT)

PET-CT can be used for imaging tumour response to therapy. Most studies suggest FDG PET has a high specificty but low sensitivity for detecting recurrent disease and is inferior to CT in detecting small tumour recurrence. Recent studies have demonstrated high sensitivity and a positive predictive value in identifying potentially resectable recurrent ovarian cancer with negative CT findings.[7]

Colonoscopy and mammography

Those exclude a primary colonic or breast lesion with ovarian metastasis.

Laparoscopy

It can be used in the management of an ovarian mass at moderate/high risk for malignancy.[4]

Treatment

Stages I and II have 5-year survival rates of 79–87% and 57–67%, respectively, while stages III and IV have 5-year survival rates that vary from 11 to 41%. The cornerstone of treatment of ovarian cancer is surgery.

Platinum-based chemotherapy is often initially efficacious in epithelial ovarian cancer. Currently, carboplatin and a taxane are considered the standard of care. For instance, carboplatin at 5.0–7.5 area under the plasma concentration–time curve and 175 mg/m^2 of paclitaxel infused over 3 h or 75 mg/m^2 of cisplatin and 135 mg/m2 of paclitaxel infused over 24 h are used. The treatment of early stage epithelial ovarian cancer is controversial. Adjuvant carboplatin/paclitaxel for three cycles versus six cycles in women with completely resected stage IC and II or clear cell or poorly differentiated stage IA and IB epithelial ovarian cancer is being compared by Gynecologic Oncology Group (GOG)157. The final data has not been published.[8]

Advanced epithelial ovarian cancer involves six cycles of either of the above regimens. GOG158 demonstrated that, while equivalent in efficacy, the combination of carboplatin/paclitaxel is preferable to cisplatin/paclitaxel due to its superior toxicity profile. Neoadjuvant chemotherapy followed by optimal debulking may be considered to be a safe and valuable treatment alternative in patients with primarily unresectable advanced stage bulky ovarian cancer.[4]

Recurrent ovarian cancer treatment is dependent upon the nature of the recurrence, the timing of the recurrence, the prior adjuvant chemotherapy used and the response to the prior regimen.[8]

When tumours of low malignant potential or borderline tumours are diagnosed in younger women at stage 1, the 5-year survival rate is 80%. Microscopic invasion influences the survival. Treatment includes cytoreductive surgery and comprehensive staging.

Follow-up

Surveillance of epithelial ovarian cancer consists of a physical examination and evaluation of serial serum tumour markers (e.g. CA125). Conventional helical CT imaging, using both oral and intravenous contrast, is obtained depending on the symptoms or with rising serum CA125 level.[9]

References

1. Barnholtz-Sloan JS, Schwartz AG, Qureshi F, Jacques S, Malone J, Munkarah AR. Ovarian cancer: changes in patterns at diagnosis and relative survival over the last three decades. *Am J Obstet Gynecol* 2003; **189**: 1120–7.
2. Ozlos R (editor). *Atlas of Clinical Oncology Ovarian Cancer*. American Cancer Society; 2003.
3. Disaia PJ, Bloss JD. Treatment of ovarian cancer: new strategies. *Gynecol Oncol* 2003; **90**: S39–44.
4. Jacobs J, Shepherd JH, Oram DH *et al.* (editors). *Ovarian Cancer*. 2002.
5. Kurjak A, Kupesic S, Sparac V, Prka M, Bekavac I. The detection of stage I ovarian cancer by three-dimensional sonography and power Doppler. *Gynecol Oncol* 2003; **90**(2): 258–64.
6. Cho SM, Ha HK, Byun JY *et al.* Usefulness of FDG PET for assessment of early recurrent epithelial ovarian cancer. *Am J Roentgenol* 2002; **179**: 391–5.
7. Bristow RE, Del Carmen MG, Pannu HK *et al.* Clinically occult recurrent ovarian cancer: patient selection for secondary cytoreductive surgery using combined PET/CT. *Gynecol Oncol* 2003; **90**: 519–28.
8. Hoskins W, Perez CA, Young RC. Principles and Practice of Gynecologic Oncology. 2000.
9. Spriggs D. Optimal sequencing in treatment of recurrent ovarian cancer. *Gynecol Oncol* 2003; **90**: S39–44.

OVARIAN CANCER

† The FIGO staging system

FIGO Stage	1	IA	IB	IC	II	IIA	IIB	IIC
	Carcinoma is strictly confined to the ovary	Growth limited to one ovary: no ascites present containing malignant cells, no tumour on the external surface and capsule intact	Growth limited to both ovaries: no ascites present containing malignant cells, no tumour on the external surfaces and capsules intact	Tumour either stage Ia or Ib, but with tumour on surface of one or both ovaries or with capsule ruptured or with ascites present containing malignant cells or with positive peritoneal washings	Growth involving one or both ovaries with pelvic extension	Extension and/or metastases to the uterus and/or tubes	Extension to other pelvic tissues	Tumour either stage IIa or IIb, but with tumour on the surface of one or both ovaries or with capsule(s) ruptured or with ascites present containing malignant cells or with positive peritoneal washings

‡ American Joint Committee on Cancer surgical staging system

AJCC Stage	T	T1a	T1b	T1c	T2a	T2b	T2c
	N						
	M						

IA

IB

IC — Malignant cells in ascites/washings

IIA

IIB — Rectum, Aorta

IIC — Malignant cells in ascites/washings

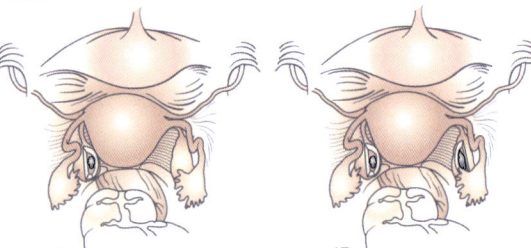

IA T1a Borderline ovarian carcinoma. The coronal reformatted contrast-enhanced CT image shows a large cystic mass (yellow arrow) above the bladder (asterisk). Some enhancing nodules (white arrow) can be seen on the wall of this lesion.

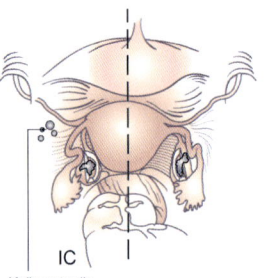

IA T1a Ovarian cystadenocarcinoma. Contrast-enhanced axial CT shows the ovarian cancer as a large complex solid cystic mass (arrows) arising out of the pelvis. No malignant cells were found in the small amount of free fluid (asterisk) seen in the pelvis.

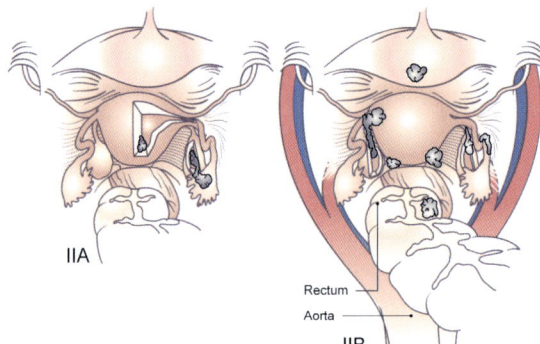

IC T1c Endometroid ovarian cancer. The contrast-enhanced CT image shows the ovarian tumour (arrow) anterior to the uterus (asterisk). Cytology from the peritoneal fluid was positive for malignant cells.

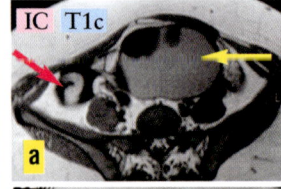
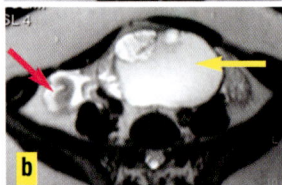

IC T1c Well-differentiated mucinous ovarian carcinoma. (a) Axial T1-weighted and (b) axial T2-weighted images show a solid cystic mass (yellow arrow) arising from the left ovary. A small amount of malignant ascites (magenta arrow) can be seen in the right iliac fossa.

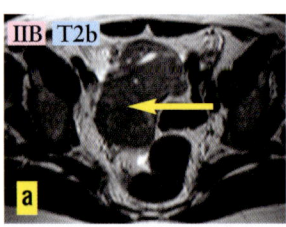
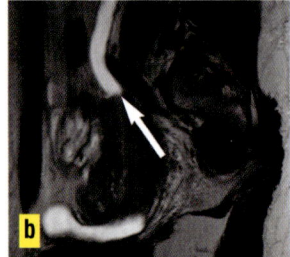

IIB T2b Poorly differentiated serous cystadenocarcinoma of the ovary. (a) Axial T2-weighted and (b) sagittal T2-weighted images show right ovarian mass invading the uterus and right Fallopian tube (yellow arrow). It extends to the pelvic side wall where it is obstructing the lower end of the right ureter (white arrow).

(Images courtesy of Dr JC Healy, Chelsea and Westminster Hospital)

III

Tumour involving one or both ovaries with histologically confirmed peritoneal implants outside the pelvis and/or positive retroperitoneal or inguinal nodes: superficial liver metastases equal stage III and tumour is limited to the true pelvis, but with histological proven malignant extension to the small bowel or omentum

IIIA

Tumour grossly limited to the true pelvis, with negative nodes, but with histologically confirmed microscopic seeding of abdominal peritoneal surfaces or histologically proven extension to the small bowel or mesentery

IIIB

Tumour of one or both ovaries with histologically confirmed implants, peritoneal metastasis of abdominal peritoneal surfaces and none exceeding 2 cm in diameter: nodes are negative

IIIC

Peritoneal metastasis beyond the pelvis >2 cm in diameter and/or positive retroperitoneal or inguinal nodes

IIIC *cont.–* **IV**

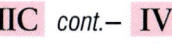

T3a

T3b

T3c   **any T**
              N1

T3c *cont.–* **M1**

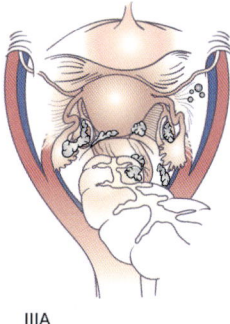

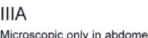

IIIA
Microscopic only in abdomen

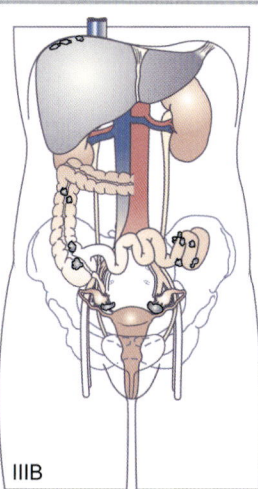

IIIB

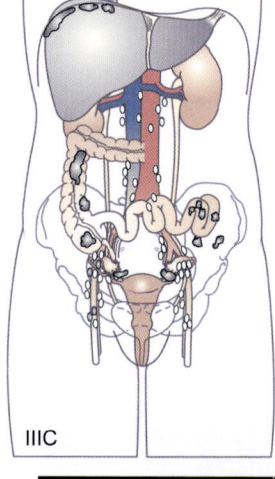

IIIC

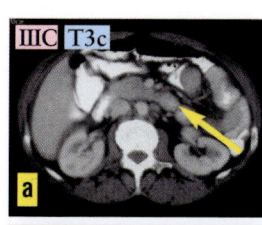

Cystadenocarcinoma of the ovary with malignant lymph nodes. Axial CT images through (a) the abdomen and (b) the pelvis show para-aortic and pelvic adenopathy (yellow arrow) and a large complex mass (magenta arrow) anterior to the uterus (asterisk).

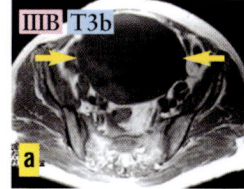

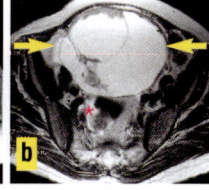

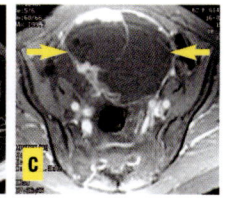

Poorly differentiated serous cystadenocarcinoma of the ovary. (a) Axial T1-weighted, (b) axial T2-weighted and (c) axial gadolinium-enhanced, fat-suppressed T1-weighted images show a complex solid cystic ovarian mass (arrows). Trace amounts of fluid can be seen in the pelvis (asterisk). Peritoneal metastases (<1 cm) could not be seen on imaging.

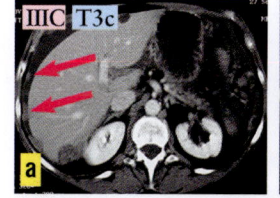

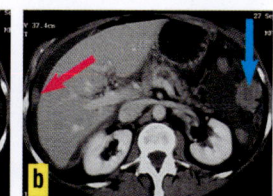

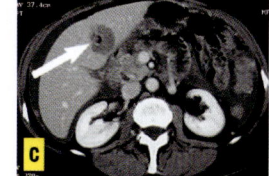

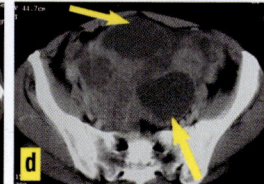

Serous cystadenocarcinoma of the ovary. Axial sections through (a)–(c) the abdomen and (d) the pelvis show a large pelvis mass (yellow arrows) and disease in the peritoneum and omental involvement. Nodular deposits can be seen on the diaphram (magenta arrow), falciform ligament (white arrow) and omentum (blue arrow).

† The FIGO staging system

I – IIIC (start)

←

IIIC

Peritoneal metastasis beyond the pelvis >2 cm in diameter and/or positive retroperitoneal or inguinal nodes

IV

Growth involving one or both ovaries with distant metastases: if pleural effusion is present, there must be positive cytology to allot a case to stage IV – parenchymal liver metastasis equals stage IV

‡ American Joint Committee on Cancer surgical staging system

T1a – T3c (start)

←

T3c **any T**
N1

any T
any N
M1

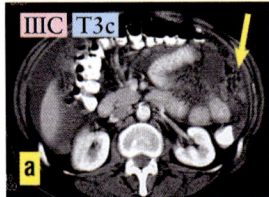
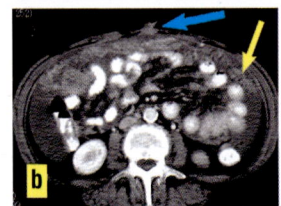
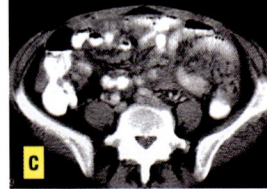
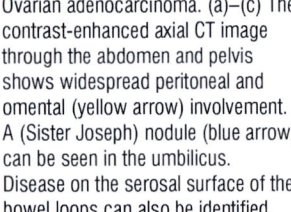

Ovarian adenocarcinoma. (a)–(c) The contrast-enhanced axial CT image through the abdomen and pelvis shows widespread peritoneal and omental (yellow arrow) involvement. A (Sister Joseph) nodule (blue arrow) can be seen in the umbilicus. Disease on the serosal surface of the bowel loops can also be identified.

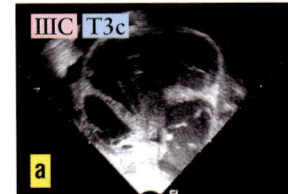
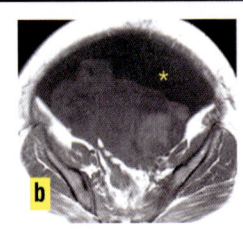
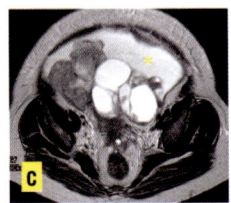
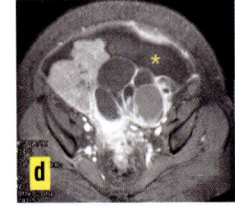

Poorly differentiated endometroid cancer. (a) Transverse section from a transvaginal ultrasound (courtesy of Dr J. A. W. Webb) shows a solid cystic mass with free fluid in the pelvis. (b) Axial T1-weighted, (c) axial T2-weighted and (d) axial gadolinium-enhanced, fat-suppressed T1-weighted images show a large solid cystic mass (arrows) and ascites (asterisk).

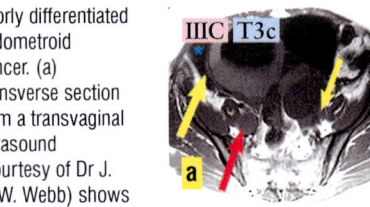
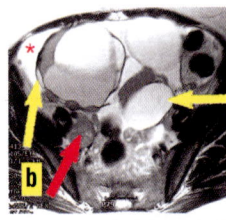
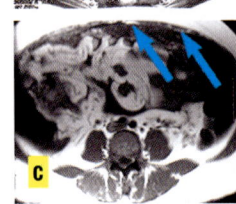

Ovarian cancer. (a) Axial T1-weighted and (b) axial T2-weighted scans through the pelvis show a large mass (yellow arrows). Free fluid (asterisk) and lymph nodes (magenta arrows) can be seen in the pelvis. (c) An axial T1-weighted section through the abdomen shows omental thickening (blue arrows).

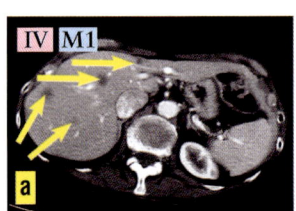
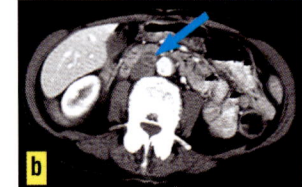
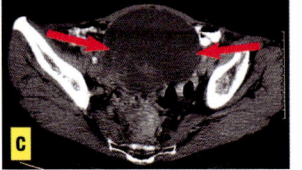

Ovarian cancer with liver metastases. (a)–(c) Contrast-enhanced CT scans show multiple liver lesions (yellow arrows), aorta-caval adenopathy (blue arrow) and the ovarian cancer (magenta arrows) in the pelvis.

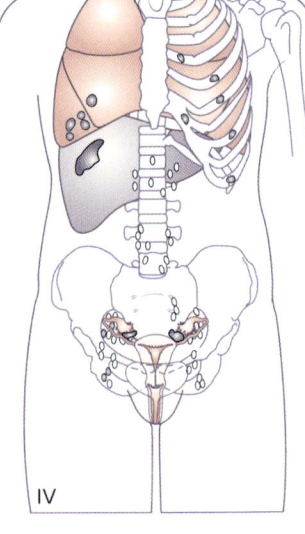

IV

GESTATIONAL TROPHOBLASTIC DISEASE

K. Sieunarine, J.R. Smith, A. Aylwin and A. Mitchell

Introduction

Gestational trophoblastic disease (GTD) includes a spectrum of cellular proliferation of trophoblasts ranging from the various forms of hydatidiform mole (complete and partial) through invasive moles and the malignant trophoblastic tumours choriocarcinomas to placental site trophoblastic tumours (PSTTs). Gestational trophoblastic tumour (GTT) is the term used for denoting those conditions that require more active intervention, usually chemotherapy and includes invasive moles, choriocarcinomas and placental site tumours.

Staging

An accurate staging and classification system for GTD will enable clinicians to assess the prognosis or risk of patients and to individualize and optimize their treatment. To date there has been a variety of staging and classification systems used by different treatment centres, which has made meaningful comparison of treatment results and the evaluation of new treatment protocols difficult.

Staging should be based on history, clinical examination and appropriate laboratory and radiological studies. Since urinary human chorionic gonadotrophin (hCG) and serum bhCG titres accurately reflect clinical disease, histological verification is not required for diagnosis, although it may aid in therapy.

The classic anatomical staging system for GTD1 of the International Federation of Gynecology and Obstetrics (Federation Internationale Gynecologique Obstetrique or FIGO) describes stage I as disease confined to the uterus and stage II as disease that extends outside of the uterus, but is limited to the genital structures (adnexa, vagina and broad ligament). Stage III refers to disease that extends to the lungs with or without genital tract involvement and stage _V to disease at other metastatic sites (e.g. the liver and brain).

The FIGO Oncology Committee accepted a new revised classification of GTD in March 2002.2 This combined the classic FIGO anatomical staging system with a revised World Health Organization risk factor scoring system3 (see Table 1).

In order to stage and allot a risk factor score, a patient's diagnosis is allocated to a stage as represented by a Roman numeral I to IV (Table 7.1). This is then separated from the sum of all the actual risk factor scores by a colon (Table 7.2), e.g. stage FIGO IV: 13. For the purposes of reporting patients are divided into high-risk (score of ≥7) and low-risk (score of 0–6) groups.

PSTTs and their non-malignant counterparts are excluded.

Principal Investigations

Histopathology

This will normally be available for patients who have had a molar pregnancy and in most cases of non-molar pregnancies.

Human chorionic gonadotrophin estimations

This provides the key to monitoring the activity of the disease, its response to treatment and follow-up.

Ultrasound

Ultrasound with Doppler assessment should be routine in managing these patients. In the pelvis the uterine size and volume can be measured, which may provide an important potential prognostic variable.[4] Doppler ultrasound can assess the vascularity of the disease. A low pulsatility index in the uterine arteries (as measured by Doppler ultrasound) correlates with the development of drug resistance in the tumour.[4] One study confirmed that, if the pulsatility index in the uterine arteries is <1, this significantly correlates with the development of resistance to methotrexate chemotherapy in low-risk patients.[5] The liver should also be scanned for

Table 7.1. **Classic FIGO staging system for GTD**

FIGO Stage	Description
I	Disease confined to the uterus
II	Disease extends outside of the uterus but is limited to the genital structures (adnexa, vagina and broad ligament)
III	Disease extends to the lungs with or without known genital tract involvement
IV	Disease at other metastatic sites

Table 7.2. **FIGO/WHO risk factor scoring system for GTD**

FIGO risk factor scoring values	0	1	2	4
Age (years)	<40	≥ 40	ñ	ñ
Antecedent pregnancy	Mole	Abortion	Term	–
Interval from index pregnancy (months)	<4	4 ñ <7	7 ñ <13	≥ 13
Pre-treatment serum hCG (IU/l)	$<10^3$	$10^3 - <10^4$	$10^4 - <10^5$	$≥ 10^5$
Largest tumour size (including uterus) (cm)	<3	3 ñ <5	≥ 5	ñ
Site of metastases	Lung	Spleen, kidney	Gastrointestinal	Liver, brain
Number of metastases	–	1 – 4	5 – 8	>8
Previous failed chemotherapy	–	–	Single drug	Two or more drugs

Principal investigations *continued*

hepatic metastases. Theca lutein cyst size and persistence correlate with the development of post-molar GTD.

Chest X-ray

Chest X-ray is appropriate for diagnosing lung metastases (for example, from invasive moles or choriocarcinomas). Low-risk patients are usually managed on the basis of a chest X-ray. It is the chest X-ray that is used for counting the number of lung metastases to evaluate the risk factor score not the computed tomography (CT) scan (see page 29).

Computed tomographic scanning

Although CT scanning of the chest is more sensitive than a chest X-ray, the whole body is not routinely CT scanned unless there are clinical indications, e.g. headache. In high-risk patients the delineation of metastatic disease sites (intra-abdominal, lung, liver and brain) by CT scanning is important in determining management.

Magnetic resonance imaging scanning

Magnetic resonance imaging (MRI) is the investigation of choice if central nervous system (CNS) metastases are suspected. MRI should be performed if cerebral metastases are suspected, even when the CT scan is normal. MRI detects lesions missed on a CT scan, particularly in the posterior fossa. MRI can play a role in management for determining tumour involvement of the great vessels and urinary and gastrointestianl tracts, before possible surgery.

Lumbar puncture

Patients with pulmonary disease are at risk of developing brain metastases and some oncologists find hCG estimations of the cerebrospinal fluid very useful in detecting metastatic disease when the scans are normal.[6]

One of the main reasons for current treatment success is the inherent chemosensitivity of GTD and GTTs.

Given its efficacy and safety profile, methotrexate/folinic acid remains the treatment of choice for low-risk patients (see Table 2)

For relapsed patients (high risk) or with disease resistant to EMA/CO (actinomycin D, etoposide and methotrexate/vincristine (oncovin) and cyclophosphamide), the EP/EMA regime is used, which is etoposide and cisplatin alternating weekly with methotrexate, actinomycin D and etoposide (see Table 2). The development of drug resistance is one of the main causes of treatment failure.

Surgery can be an important component of salvage treatment and often may be clearly therapeutic. Surgery plays an important role in the primary treatment of patients with PSTTs since PSTTs have rather variable chemosensitivity. Hysterectomy is the treatment of choice for PSTTs limited to the uterus.

The role of radiotherapy is uncertain: however, there is a role for stereotaxic radiotherapy in the occasional case where there is a single site of relapse.

After completion of chemotherapy patients are monitored by serial hCG estimations. CT and MRI scanning allow better localization of sites of resistant disease. MRI is suitable for disease within the pelvis and brain whilst CT scanning is appropriate for the chest and abdomen.

Table 3. **Treatment for low-risk patients**

Low-risk cases[a]		*Low-risk disease resistant to methotrexate*	
Days[b]	**Treatment**	**Serum bhCG**	**Treatment**
e.g. 1, 3, 5 and 7	Methotrexate	~100 IU/l	Actinomycin D
e.g. 2, 4, 6 and 8	Folinic acid	>100 IU/l	EMA/CO

[a]Cycles are repeated (e.g. after a 6-day drug-free interval) depending on the regimen used.
[b]Many alternatives possible.

Table 4. **Treatment for high-risk patients**

	Week 1	*Week 2[a]*
Day	**Treatment**	
1	EMA	CO
2	Actinomycin D, etoposide (as before) and folinic acid 24 h after methotrexate commenced	

[a]The response to chemotherapy is monitored by serial βhCG estimations.

References

1. FIGO Oncology Committee Report. *Int J Gynecol Obstet* 1992; **39**: 149–50.
2. Ngan HY. The FIGO staging for gestational trophoblastic neoplasia 2000, FIGO Committee Report. *Int J Gynecol Obstet* 2002; **77**: 285–7.
3. Kohorn EI, Goldstein DP, Hancock BW *et al.* Combining the staging system of the International Federation of Gynecology and Obstetrics with the scoring system of the World Health Organization for trophoblastic neoplasia. Report of the Working Committee of the International Society for the Study of Trophoblastic Disease and the International Gynecologic Cancer Society. *Int J Gynecol Cancer* 2000; **10**: 84–8.
4. Long MG, Boultbee JE, Langley R *et al.* Doppler assessment of the uterine circulation and its relationship to the clinical behaviour of gestational trophoblastic tumours requiring chemotherapy. *Br J Cancer* 1992; **66**: 883–7.
5. Agarwal R, Srrickland S, McNeish IA *et al.* Doppler ultrasonography of the uterine artery and the response to chemotherapy in patients with gestational trophoblastic tumors. *Clin Cancer Res* 2002; **8**: 1142–7.
6. Bagshawe KD, Harland S. Immunodiagnosis and monitoring of gonadotrophin producing metastases in the central nervous system. *Cancer* 1976; **38**: 112–18.

Further reading

Hancock BW, Newlands ES, Berkowitz RS, Cole LA (editors). *Gestational Trophoblastic Disease,* 2nd edn. International Society for the Study of Trophoblastic Diseases; 2003.

Ngan HYS, Odicino F, Maisonneuve P *et al.* Gestational trophoblastic diseases. *J Epidemiol Biostat* 2001; **6**(1): 175–84.

Smith JR, Del Priore G, Curtin J, Monaghan JM (editors). *An Atlas of Gynecologic Oncology* 2nd edn. Taylor & Francis; 2005.

GESTATIONAL TROPHOBLASTIC DISEASE

	I	+the sum of **FIGO risk factor scoring values**	**0**	**1**	**2**	**4**		**II**	+the sum of **FIGO risk factor scoring values**
FIGO Stage	Disease confined to the uterus	Age (years)	<40	≥ 40	ñ	ñ		Disease extends outside of the uterus but is limited to the genital structures (adnexa, vagina and broad ligament)	
		Antecedent pregnancy	Mole	Abortion	Term	–			
		Interval from index pregnancy (months)	<4	4 ñ <7	7 ñ <13	≥ 13			
		Pre-treatment serum hCG (IU/l)	$<10^3$	$10^3 - <10^4$	$10^4 - <10^5$	$\geq 10^5$			
		Largest tumour size (including uterus) (cm)	<3	3 ñ <5	≥ 5	ñ			
		Site of metastases	Lung	Spleen and kidney	Gastrointestinal	Liver and brain			
		Number of metastases	–	1 – 4	5 – 8	>8			
		Previous failed chemotherapy	–	–	Single drug	Two or more drugs			

AJCC T Stage M	**T1** No risk factors	**T1** One risk factor	**T1** Two risk factors	**T2** No risk factors	**T2** One risk factor

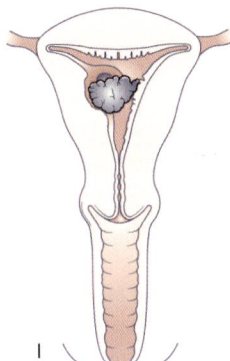

I

TNM definitions

Primary tumour (T).
T1: disease limited to the uterus.
T2: disease outside of the uterus but is limited to genital structures (the ovary, tube, vagina and broad ligaments).

Regional Lymph Nodes (N)
There is no regional nodal designation (N classification) in the staging of gestational trophoblastic tumors. Nodal involvement in these tumors is rare but has an extremely poor prognosis. Nodal metastases should be classified as metastatic M1b disease

Distant metastasis (M)
M1a: Lung metastasis
M1b: All other distant metastasis

Risk factors affecting staging include the following:
1. hCG > 100,000 IU/24-hour urine.
2. The detection of disease more than 6 months from termination of the antecedent pregnancy

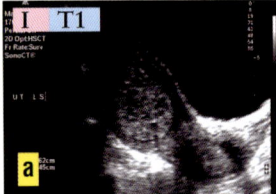
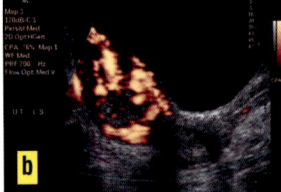

Longitudinal ultrasound sections of the pelvis showing a large heterogenous echogenic tumour confined to the uterus (stage I). (a) Grey scale image and (b) power Doppler image demonstrating marked vascularity of the tumour.

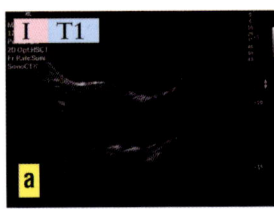
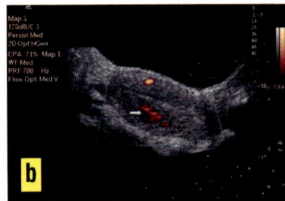

Longitudinal ultrasound sections of the pelvis. (a) Non-visible tumour and (b) power Doppler image showing the increased vascularity of a small stage I isoechoic lesion (arrow).

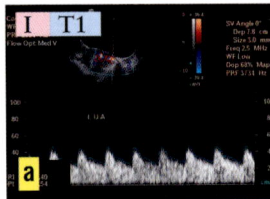

Transverse ultrasound image with colour Doppler of the uterus in a patient with a stage I tumour, with pulse wave Doppler of the left uterine artery demonstrating a low (<1.0) pulsatility index (PI = peak systolic – diastolic velocity/mean) due to the reduced end organ resistance characteristic of gestational trophoblastic tumours.

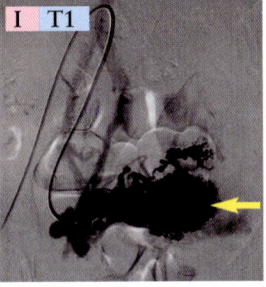

Digital subtraction angiogram of the pelvis with a catheter in the right uterine artery showing the significant vascularity of a stage I tumour (arrow), secondary to neoangiogenesis.

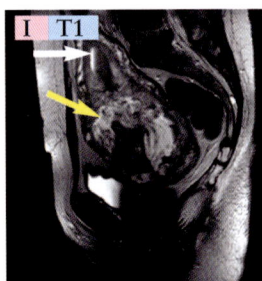

Sagittal T2-weighted image of the pelvis in a patient with a large heterogeneous stage I uterine tumour (yellow arrow). Note fluid within the obstructed endometrial cavity (white arrow).

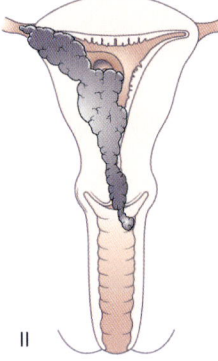

II

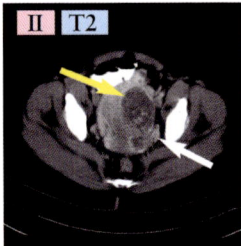

Axial CT image of the pelvis showing a large heterogeneous left-sided uterine mass (yellow arrow) extending along the broad ligament to the left ovary (white arrow) (stage II).

III +the sum of **FIGO risk factor scoring values**

Disease extends to
the lungs with or
without known
genital tract
involvement

IV +the sum of **FIGO risk factor scoring values**

Disease at other
metastatic sites

T2	**T3**	**T3**	**T3**	**any T**	**any T**	**any T**
Two risk factors	**M1a**	**M1a**	**M1a**	**M1b**	**M1b**	**M1b**
	No risk factors	One risk factor	Two risk factors	No risk factors	One risk factor	Two risk factors

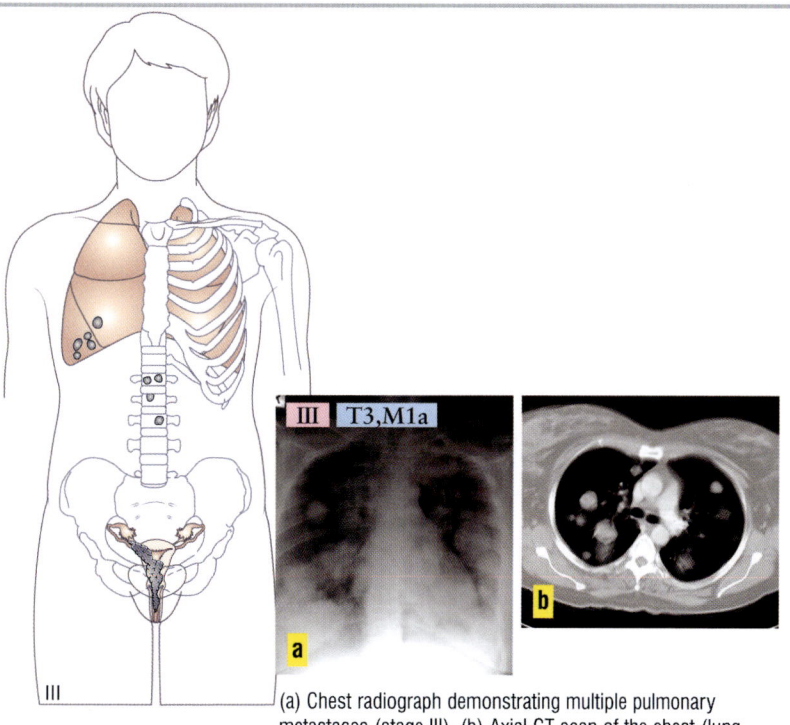

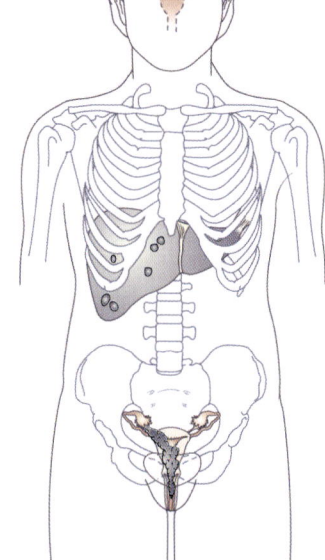

III **T3,M1a**

b

a

(a) Chest radiograph demonstrating multiple pulmonary metastases (stage III). (b) Axial CT scan of the chest (lung windows) of the same patient.

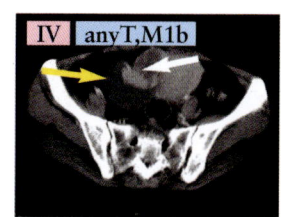

IV **anyT,M1b**

Axial CT scan of the pelvis showing a heterogeneous mass (arrowhead) arising from the uterus and invading the bladder (arrow) (stage IV tumour).

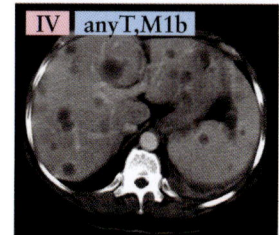

IV **anyT,M1b**

Intravenous contrast-enhanced CT of the liver demonstrating multiple hypoattenuating hepatic and splenic metastases (stage IV).

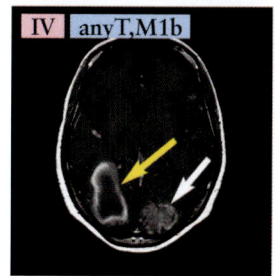

IV **anyT,M1b**

Gadolinium-enhanced axial T1-weighted MRI of the brain showing two metastases, one cystic and rim enhancing (arrow) and the other solid and heterogeneously enhancing (arrowhead) (stage IV).

Printed in Thailand